Sleep in the Elderly

Editors

MARGARITA OKS
STEVEN H. FEINSILVER

CLINICS IN
GERIATRIC MEDICINE

www.geriatric.theclinics.com

August 2021 • Volume 37 • Number 3

ELSEVIER

1600 John F. Kennedy Boulevard • Suite 1800 • Philadelphia, Pennsylvania, 19103-2899

http://www.theclinics.com

CLINICS IN GERIATRIC MEDICINE Volume 37, Number 3
August 2021 ISSN 0749–0690, ISBN-13: 978-0-323-79597-5

Editor: Katerina Heidhausen
Developmental Editor: Ann Gielou M. Posedio

Clinics in Geriatric Medicine (ISSN 0749-0690) is published quarterly by Elsevier Inc., 360 Park Avenue South, New York, NY 10010-1710. Months of issue are February, May, August, and November. Business and Editorial Offices: 1600 John F. Kennedy Blvd., Suite 1800, Philadelphia, PA 191023-2899. Periodicals postage paid at New York, NY, and additional mailing offices. Subscription prices are $295.00 per year (US individuals), $875.00 per year (US institutions), $100.00 per year (US & Canadian student/resident), $320.00 per year (Canadian individuals), $928.00 per year (Canadian institutions), $418.00 per year (international individuals), $928.00 per year (international institutions), and $195.00 per year (international student/resident). Foreign air speed delivery is included in all *Clinics* subscription prices. All prices are subject to change without notice. POSTMASTER: Send address changes to *Clinics in Geriatric Medicine,* Elsevier Health Sciences Division, Subscription Customer Service, 3251 Riverport Lane, Maryland Heights, MO 63043. **Telephone: 1-800-654-2452 (U.S. and Canada); 314-447-8871 (outside U.S. and Canada). Fax: 314-447-8029. E-mail:** journalscustomerservice-usa@elsevier.com **(for print support) or** journalsonlinesupport-usa@elsevier.com **(for online support).**

Reprints. For copies of 100 or more, of articles in this publication, please contact the Commercial Reprints Department, Elsevier Inc., 360 Park Avenue South, New York, New York 10010-1710. Tel.: 212-633-3874; Fax: 212-633-3820, E-mail: reprints@elsevier.com.

Clinics in Geriatric Medicine is covered in *MEDLINE/PubMed (Index Medicus), EMBASE/Excerpta Medica, Current Contents/Clinical Medicine (CC/CM),* and the *Cumulative Index to Nursing & Allied Health Literature.*

Contributors

EDITORS

MARGARITA OKS, MD
Associate Program Director, Pulmonary and Critical Care Medicine, Associate Director, Center for Sleep Medicine, Assistant Professor of Medicine, Division of Pulmonary, Critical Care and Sleep Medicine, Donald and Barbara Zucker School of Medicine at Hofstra/Northwell, Lenox Hill Hospital, New York, New York

STEVEN H. FEINSILVER, MD
Director, Center for Sleep Medicine, Professor of Medicine, Donald and Barbara Zucker School of Medicine at Hofstra/Northwell, Lenox Hill Hospital, New York, New York

AUTHORS

DEREK J. CHONG, MD, MSc
Vice Chair, Department of Neurology, Assistant Professor, Donald and Barbara Zucker School of Medicine at Hofstra/Northwell, Lenox Hill Hospital, New York, New York

JOSEPH A. DIAMOND, MD
Associate Professor of Medicine, Donald and Barbara Zucker School of Medicine at Hofstra/Northwell, Director of Nuclear Cardiology, Department of Cardiology, Long Island Jewish Hospital, Northwell Health, New Hyde Park, New York

MATTHEW R. EBBEN, PhD
Associate Professor of Psychology in Clinical Neurology, Weill Medical College of Cornell University, Center for Sleep Medicine, New York, New York; Polysomnographic Technology Training Program, Kingsborough Community College (CUNY), Brooklyn, New York

STEVEN H. FEINSILVER, MD
Director, Center for Sleep Medicine, Professor of Medicine, Donald and Barbara Zucker School of Medicine at Hofstra/Northwell, Lenox Hill Hospital, New York, New York

STELLA S. HAHN, MD
Assistant Professor, Division of Pulmonary, Critical Care and Sleep Medicine, Department of Medicine, Donald and Barbara Zucker School of Medicine at Hofstra/Northwell, Great Neck, New York

OKI ISHIKAWA, MD
Department of Pulmonary and Critical Care, Fellow, Donald and Barbara Zucker School of Medicine at Hofstra/Northwell, Lenox Hill Hospital, New York, New York

HAISAM ISMAIL, MD
Assistant Professor of Medicine, Donald and Barbara Zucker School of Medicine at Hofstra/Northwell, Electrophysiologist, Department of Cardiology, Long Island Jewish Hospital, Northwell Health, New Hyde Park, New York

MAKSIM KOROTUN, DO
Assistant Professor, Division of Pulmonary, Critical Care and Sleep Medicine, Department of Medicine, Donald and Barbara Zucker School of Medicine at Hofstra/Northwell, Great Neck, New York

ANA C. KRIEGER, MD, MPH
Departments of Medicine, Neurology and Genetic Medicine, Weill Cornell Medicine/NewYork-Presbyterian Hospital, New York, New York

BECKY X. LOU, MD
Northwell Sleep Medicine Fellowship, Division of Pulmonary, Critical Care and Sleep Medicine, Department of Medicine, Donald and Barbara Zucker School of Medicine at Hofstra/Northwell, New Hyde Park, New York

MARGARITA OKS, MD
Associate Program Director, Pulmonary and Critical Care Medicine, Associate Director, Center for Sleep Medicine, Assistant Professor of Medicine, Division of Pulmonary, Critical Care and Sleep Medicine, Donald and Barbara Zucker School of Medicine at Hofstra/Northwell, Lenox Hill Hospital, New York, New York

ARPAN PATEL, MD
Department of Neurology, Donald and Barbara Zucker School of Medicine at Hofstra/Northwell, Northwell Health, Manhasset, New York

LUIS QUINTERO, DO, MPH
Assistant Professor, Division of Pulmonary, Critical Care and Sleep Medicine, Department of Medicine, Donald and Barbara Zucker School of Medicine at Hofstra/Northwell, Great Neck, New York

MARIA V. SUURNA, MD
Department of Otolaryngology, Head and Neck Surgery, Weill Cornell Medicine/NewYork-Presbyterian Hospital, New York, New York

Contents

Preface: Sleep in the Elderly: A Common and Growing Problem   ix

Margarita Oks and Steven H. Feinsilver

Normal and Abnormal Sleep in the Elderly   377

Steven H. Feinsilver

Sleep-related complaints are so common in older adults that it may be difficult to distinguish whether the complaint is a consequence of normal aging or a disease process. The elderly are more likely to have common medical problems that affect sleep, and the most common sleep problems, including sleep apnea and insomnia, are more prevalent in this demographic. This article briefly describes normal sleep in general, the clinical assessment of sleep complaints, and expected changes with aging, with an overview of the epidemiology of insomnia and sleep apnea in this age group.

Insomnia: Behavioral Treatment in the Elderly   387

Matthew R. Ebben

Sleep quality in elderly individuals is affected by increased mental and physical health issues associated with aging, but also a decrease in sleep drive and an advance of the circadian phase. These issues may, in part, be due to lifestyle changes in older adults, such as retirement and/or reduced social and physical activity, which can lead to spending more time in bed, resulting in chronic insomnia. Cognitive behavioral therapy for insomnia has been shown to be an effective treatment method for difficulty sleeping in elderly individuals and should be the first-line treatment due to its efficacy and safety profile.

Insomnia: Pharmacologic Treatment   401

Becky X. Lou and Margarita Oks

Insomnia afflicts many geriatric patients worldwide and results in both clinical and economic consequences. Prescribing hypnotics to the elderly is particularly challenging due to multitudes of adverse effects and drug interactions. Although benzodiazepines and "Z" drugs such as zolpidem have been popular in the past, they carry a high risk of adverse effects in the elderly, such as devastating falls and injuries as well as potentially an increase in mortality. Newer classes of hypnotics such as dual orexin receptor antagonists are much better tolerated and can be explored as a potential treatment for insomnia in the elderly.

Obstructive Sleep Apnea: Treatment with Positive Airway Pressure   417

Steven H. Feinsilver

As in other adults, continuous positive airway pressure treatment for obstructive sleep apnea should be the mainstay of treatment. Benefits include improvements in sleepiness and quality of life, as well as improvements in hypertension control, arrhythmias, cardiovascular risk, and mortality. This article discusses issues in prescribing this treatment, including those related specifically to elderly individuals.

Obstructive Sleep Apnea: Non–positive Airway Pressure Treatments   429

Maria V. Suurna and Ana C. Krieger

Undiagnosed and untreated obstructive sleep apnea (OSA) is associated with health comorbidities and negatively affects quality of life. Alternative treatments should be considered in patients who are unable to tolerate or benefit from positive airway pressure treatment. When properly indicated, positional devices, oral appliances, airway surgery, and hypoglossal nerve stimulation have been shown to be effective in treating OSA. Hypoglossal nerve stimulation is a successful second-line treatment with low associated morbidity and complication rate.

Obstructive Sleep Apnea and Cardiovascular Disease   445

Joseph A. Diamond and Haisam Ismail

Obstructive sleep apnea (OSA) presents as repetitive interruptions of ventilation >10 seconds during sleep as a result of upper airway obstruction resulting in increased respiratory effort. Intermittent hypoxia causes physiologic changes resulting in increased catecholamine production, increased total peripheral resistance, tachycardia, and increased venous return, leading to increased cardiac output, hypertension, tachyarrhythmias, left ventricular hypertrophy, and heart failure. OSA causes an abnormal dip on 24-hour ambulatory blood pressure monitoring. Definitive diagnosis is made by polysomnography. Continuous positive airway pressure (CPAP) remains the first-line treatment. Effective treatment using CPAP reduces blood pressure and is indispensable for proper management of atrial fibrillation.

Obstructive Sleep Apnea: Cognitive Outcomes   457

Arpan Patel and Derek J. Chong

There is a strong association between obstructive sleep apnea (OSA) and cognitive dysfunction. Executive function, attention, verbal/visual long-term memory, visuospatial/constructional ability, and information processing are more likely to be affected, whereas language, psychomotor function, and short-term memory are less likely to be affected. Increased accumulation of Aß $_2$-amyloid in the brain, episodic hypoxemia, oxidative stress, vascular inflammation, and systemic comorbidities may contribute to the pathogenesis. Patients with OSA should have cognitive screening or formal testing, and patients with cognitive decline should have testing for OSA. Treatment with continuous positive airway pressure may improve cognitive symptoms in the patient with OSA.

Central Sleep Apnea   469

Oki Ishikawa and Margarita Oks

Central sleep apnea (CSA) is characterized by intermittent repetitive cessation and/or decreased breathing without effort caused by an abnormal ventilatory drive. Although less prevalent than obstructive sleep apnea, it is frequently encountered. CSA can be primary (idiopathic) or secondary in association with Cheyne-Stokes respiration, drug-induced, medical conditions such as chronic renal failure, or high-altitude periodic breathing. Risk factors have been proposed, including gender, age, heart failure, opioid use, stroke, and other chronic medical conditions. This article discusses the prevalence of CSA in the general population and within each of these at-risk populations, and clinical presentation, diagnostic methods, and treatment.

Rapid Eye Movement Behavior Disorder and Other Parasomnias   483

Maksim Korotun, Luis Quintero, and Stella S. Hahn

Rapid eye movement (REM) behavior disorder (RBD) is characterized by loss of skeletal muscle atonia that can lead to dream enactment. This condition can cause harm to patients and their bed partners if appropriate safety measures are not ensured. This condition is often the initial presenting symptom in a group of complex neurodegenerative processes. Definitive diagnosis requires a thorough history and an in-laboratory polysomnogram to look for evidence of REM sleep without atonia. Treatment options are limited but consist of sleep safety measures and pharmacotherapy. Patients diagnosed with idiopathic RBD associated with alpha-synucleinopathy are likely to have progression of disease.

CLINICS IN GERIATRIC MEDICINE

FORTHCOMING ISSUES

November 2021
Women's Health
Elizabeth Cobbs and Karen Blackstone,
Editors

February 2022
Alcohol and Substance Abuse in Older Adults
George T. Grossberg and Rita Khoury,
Editors

RECENT ISSUES

May 2021
Peripheral Nerve Disease in the Geriatric Population
Peter H. Jin, *Editor*

February 2021
Gastroenterology
Amir E. Soumekh and Philip O. Katz,
Editors

SERIES OF RELATED INTEREST

Medical Clinics of North America
Primary Care: Clinics in Office Practice

THE CLINICS ARE AVAILABLE ONLINE!
Access your subscription at:
www.theclinics.com

Preface

Sleep in the Elderly: A Common and Growing Problem

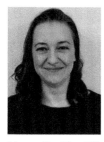 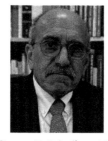

Margarita Oks, MD   Steven H. Feinsilver, MD
Editors

The elderly are the fastest growing segment of the world's population. Sleep complaints increase with aging, but it is often difficult to distinguish the effects of aging from the effects of diseases and lifestyle changes in this population. It remains unclear exactly what the expected changes in quality and quantity of sleep are in the elderly.

We have tried in this issue to review some important principles of sleep medicine for the physician caring for the elderly, emphasizing, where known, how diagnosis and treatment of common sleep problems might be different with aging. The first article reviews what is known about sleep with aging and the epidemiology of sleep diseases in this population. It is difficult to know what sleep changes should be expected in the healthy elderly, but it should not be assumed that sleep necessarily deteriorates; most sleep complaints should be evaluated and addressed in this age group about the same as in a younger population.

Insomnia is a particular challenge with aging. The treatment of insomnia should always begin with a behavioral approach, outlined in the article by Ebben. However, behavioral therapy alone is not always practical or sufficient, and the pharmacology of insomnia treatment is discussed in the article by Lou and Oks.

Obstructive sleep apnea remains the most significant disease in sleep medicine. Feinsilver reviews a practical approach to positive airway pressure (PAP) treatment. Although PAP is generally very successful, it is not always tolerated, and compliance with treatment can be difficult. Suurna and Krieger review non-PAP approaches to treating this disease.

Many patients with obstructive sleep apnea will have relatively mild symptoms of daytime sleepiness, snoring, or disturbed sleep. It is often difficult to know which patients require treatment. Much of this decision making is based on what we know about the consequences of the disease, particularly its effects on the heart and on the brain, as reviewed in the articles by Diamond and Ismail and Chong and Patel, respectively.

Clin Geriatr Med 37 (2021) ix–x
https://doi.org/10.1016/j.cger.2021.04.010
0749-0690/21/© 2021 Published by Elsevier Inc.

Ishikawa and Oks discuss central sleep apnea. Although much rarer than obstructive sleep apnea, it remains a significant clinical challenge, and treatment is currently the subject of controversy since the discovery that a previously recommended treatment may have actually increased mortality.

Finally, the most significant parasomnia in the elderly, REM sleep behavior disorder, is not rare, may be dangerous, and can be easily recognized by history. This is a very treatable disorder, which may be the earliest manifestation of progressive neurologic disease. This and other parasomnias are discussed by Korotun and colleagues.

This has been a remarkably challenging year for this or any project. Many of us have been nearly overwhelmed by the COVID-19 pandemic both professionally and personally. Several of the authors are pulmonary and/or critical care physicians who have had to put sleep medicine on hold for much of the past year. We would like to thank all of our contributors for taking the time to produce this issue, and the editorial staff at Elsevier for their patient support.

Margarita Oks, MD
Pulmonary and Critical Care Medicine
Donald & Barbara Zucker School of
Medicine at Hofstra/Northwell
Lenox Hill Hospital
100 East 77th Street
New York, NY 10075, USA

Steven H. Feinsilver, MD
Donald & Barbara Zucker School of
Medicine at Hofstra/Northwell
Lenox Hill Hospital
100 East 77th Street
New York, NY 10075, USA

E-mail addresses:
moks@northwell.edu (M. Oks)
sfeinsil@northwell.edu (S.H. Feinsilver)

Normal and Abnormal Sleep in the Elderly

Steven H. Feinsilver, MD

KEYWORDS

- Elderly • Sleep apnea • Insomnia • Epidemiology • Sleep stages
- Polysomnography • Phase advance

KEY POINTS

- Sleep is a complex phenomenon with 4 distinct stages, including 3 stages of non-rapid eye movement (REM) sleep and REM.
- Sleep architecture changes with advanced age with reduced slow-wave (deepest) sleep.
- Circadian rhythm changes with normal aging often lead to a "phase advance" with earlier bedtimes and wake times.
- Sleep complaints increase with aging because of expected physiologic changes and the effects of illness and medication.

The elderly are the fastest growing segment of the world's population. One in 6 people in Europe and North America were estimated to be over the age of 65 as of 2019, rising to 1 in 4 by 2050; The number of persons aged 80 or over is expected to triple, from 143 million in 2019 to 426 million in 2050.[1] Sleep complaints increase with aging even in the absence of disease. In 1 epidemiologic study, more than half of elderly subjects had sleep complaints.[2] Many sleep complaints are indicators of poor health, and in a 3-year follow-up of elderly subjects with sleep complaints, many had resolution of their sleep symptoms with improved health,[3] seeming to imply that bad sleep is not a necessary consequence of normal aging.

WHAT IS NORMAL SLEEP?

The terminology for describing normal human sleep in stages has changed very little since originally described by Rechtshaffen and Kales[4] more than half a century ago.

Human consciousness can be divided into 3 states: wake, non–rapid eye movement (REM) sleep, and REM sleep. In a sleep laboratory polysomnogram (ie, a sleep study), measurements of electroencephalography (EEG), muscle tone with electromyography (EMG), and eye movements are used to distinguish the stages of sleep. Respiratory

Zucker School of Medicine at Hofstra Northwell Health, Center for Sleep Medicine, Lenox Hill Hospital, New York, NY, USA
E-mail address: sfeinsil@northwell.edu

Clin Geriatr Med 37 (2021) 377–386
https://doi.org/10.1016/j.cger.2021.04.001
0749-0690/21/© 2021 Elsevier Inc. All rights reserved.

geriatric.theclinics.com

monitoring includes measuring airflow by nasal pressure transducers and/or thermistors, respiratory effort by measuring chest and abdominal movement, and oximetry. End tidal or transcutaneous CO_2 sensors may be added. Electrocardiography is recorded, and leg movements may be monitored by EMG of the anterior tibialis muscle. Video is recorded using an infrared camera and light source. Additional recordings may be made for specialized studies.

Stages of sleep are summarized in **Table 1**. EEG during quiet wakefulness is a low-amplitude mixed frequency signal with relatively high muscle tone on EMG. The predominant EEG frequency is alpha rhythm (8–12 Hz; **Fig. 1**), which occurs during relaxed wakefulness with eyes closed. Sleep onset is characterized by the disappearance of alpha activity, reduction in EMG amplitude, and often slow ("rolling") eye movements. This period is the onset of stage 1 non-REM sleep, originally termed "transitional" sleep (**Fig. 2**). During this stage, sleep is light, and the subject is easily awakened. Stage 1 sleep is not considered to have much restorative value. About half of total sleep time (TST) is stage 2, identified by sleep spindles (episodes of 12–14 Hz activity lasting 0.5–1 second) and K-complexes (biphasic waves beginning with a sharp upward deflection). Spindles and K-complexes are seen in **Fig. 3**. In stage 3 sleep, at least 20% of the tracing consists of large slow waves (delta waves). Delta waves have a frequency of 0.5 to 1.5 Hz and an amplitude of at least 75 μV. Slow-wave sleep is seen in **Fig. 4**.

REM sleep was originally referred to as "paradoxic sleep," the paradox being that the brain is active while voluntary muscles are nearly paralyzed. The EEG may be difficult to distinguish from wakefulness. "REMs" are displayed in (**Fig. 5**), and the EMG shows muscle activity at the lowest level of the night. REM is thought to be the period of greatest respiratory and cardiac instability of sleep; because of the reduced muscle tone of accessory respiratory muscles, patients with diaphragmatic dysfunction may be at particular risk.

Normal sleep consists of transitions between the 4 stages of sleep in roughly 2- to 3-hour cycles (**Table 2**). There is wide variability from night to night and among individuals. After a period of up to 20 minutes on average ("sleep latency"), sleep usually begins with stage 1 sleep. A typical cycle of 90 to 110 minutes includes variable amounts of stage 2 and 3 sleep culminating in an REM period. The time to the first REM period ("REM latency") is typically 70 to 100 minutes. Generally, more deep sleep (stage 3) is seen in the first half of the night, and more REM sleep is seen in the second half of the night. Awakenings during the night are universal, although they may not be recalled the next day if brief. The quality of sleep can be expressed as sleep efficiency (SE): the ratio of TST to time in bed (TIB), and as wake time after sleep onset. Normal SE is approximately 85% in healthy adults.

Table 1
Stages of normal sleep

Sleep Stage	Characteristics	Significance
Wakefulness	Mixed-frequency, low-amplitude EEG; may see alpha waves if relaxed, eyes closed	Awake
Stage 1	Alpha disappears, may see theta waves	Light ("transitional") sleep 5%–10% of sleep time
Stage 2	Spindles and/or K-complexes seen	About 50% of sleep time
Stage 3	Theta (slow) waves	Deepest sleep
REM	REM, EEG similar to wake, low muscle tone	Dreaming sleep

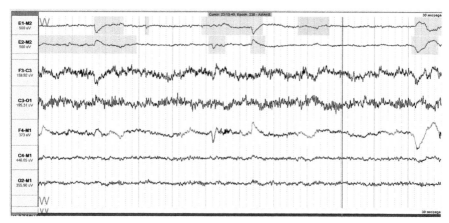

Fig. 1. Quiet wakefulness: alpha activity is prominent, seen best in central lead. All polysomnogram figures are 30-second samples. C, central; E, eye leads; F, frontal; M, mastoid; O, occipital.

WHAT IS NORMAL SLEEP IN THE ELDERLY?

Although changes appear to occur in both sleep timing and quality with aging, it is often difficult to separate normal aging from effects of both concomitant diseases and medications. The expected change in timing with aging is referred to as a "phase advance": peak sleepiness occurs earlier in the evening, normal bedtime becomes earlier, and sleep during the early morning hours is reduced. Societal pressure to keep "normal" hours may lead to elderly subjects staying awake later than optimal and becoming somewhat sleep deprived and may be one of the most important causes of poor sleep in the healthy elderly.

Common wisdom is that elderly patients need less sleep and are more likely to be sleepy during the day. The elderly do appear to get less sleep; a meta-analysis by Ohayon and colleagues[5] suggests a linear reduction in TST throughout adult life, with about 30 minutes less sleep at age 60 compared with age 40. Most studies show a reduction in SE, an increase in stage 1 (light sleep), and a reduction in stage

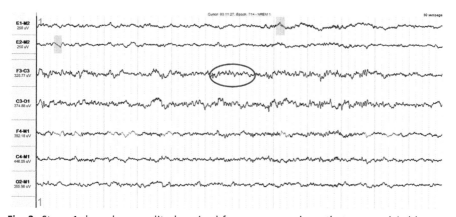

Fig. 2. Stage 1 sleep: low-amplitude, mixed-frequency, may have theta waves (*circle*).

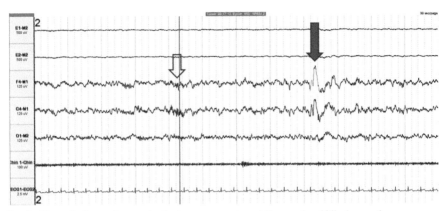

Fig. 3. Stage 2 sleep: sleep spindle (*open arrow*) and K-complex (*filled arrow*).

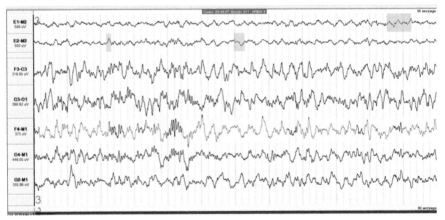

Fig. 4. Stage 3 sleep: slow (delta) waves seen in more than 20% of tracing. Here, most frontal tracing consists of slow waves.

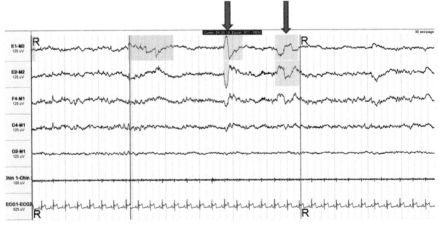

Fig. 5. REM sleep: REMs marked with arrows. EEG is mostly low-amplitude mixed-frequency, some theta.

Table 2
Normal sleep

Measurement	Definition	Normal Range
Sleep latency (SL)	Time from lights out to sleep onset	<20 min
REM latency (REML)	Time from sleep onset to first REM period	70–120 min
Total sleep time (TST)	Total time asleep	360–480 min
Time in bed (TIB)	Total time in bed attempting to sleep	Variable
Wake after sleep onset (WASO)	Time spent awake during time in bed	<15% of time in bed
Sleep efficiency (SE)	TST/TIB	>85%

3 (slow-wave sleep). Sleep latency increases only minimally, less than 10 minutes from age 20 to 80.[5] The Sleep Heart Health Study[6] showed a decline in slow-wave sleep with aging in men but not women, and a reduction in REM sleep in both men and women. In the Ohayon meta-analysis, the percentage of REM sleep as well as the time to the first REM period (REM latency) decreased with age in both men and women.

The reduction in slow-wave sleep is one of the more significant changes from adult-hood to middle age and beyond. Slow-wave sleep is considered the "deepest," most restorative stage of sleep. Normally, most growth hormone secretion occurs during slow-wave sleep. With reduced slow-wave sleep, there is a parallel reduction in growth hormone secretion, suggesting this does have physiologic significance.[7]

A summary of changes in sleep stages with aging is seen in **Table 3 Fig 6**.

The common stereotype of greater daytime sleepiness in the elderly may not be correct. One study showed a reduction in sleep propensity with aging,[8] and a study by Duffy and colleagues[9] suggests healthy elderly subjects may better tolerate sleep deprivation than younger adults.

Overall, the effect of these normal changes with aging lead to complaints of sleep maintenance more than sleep onset. As nocturnal sleep decreases, there may be more daytime sleepiness, although this is not universal, and there may be compensatory napping. However, daytime sleepiness should not be considered part of normal aging. If sleep complaints are significant, for example, affecting normal activities or cognitive functioning, or if there are other typical symptoms of a primary sleep disorder, diagnostic testing is warranted, as it would be in any other age group.

Table 3
Changes in sleep with aging

Sleep Parameter	Change
Total sleep time (TST)	Reduced
Sleep efficiency (SE)	Reduced
REM sleep	Reduced
Slow-wave sleep (SWS, stage 3)	Reduced
Sleep latency	Slightly increased
REM latency	Reduced
Wake after sleep onset (WASO)	Increased

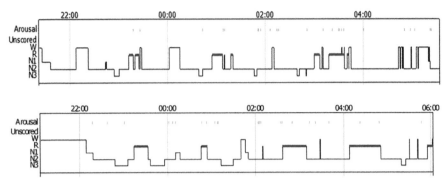

Fig. 6. Hypnograms from normal subjects. (*top*) Healthy 85-year-old. Note early sleep onset and early morning wakefulness, suggesting advanced sleep phase, several wakes, and less slow-wave sleep compared with bottom hypnogram from (*bottom*) healthy 33-year-old.

EPIDEMIOLOGY OF INSOMNIA IN THE ELDERLY
Behavioral Causes of Poor Sleep

Even in the completely healthy elderly, retirement and accompanying lifestyle changes often are accompanied by poor sleep. No longer being required to set a schedule for work may be gratifying, but a fixed schedule (and particularly a constant wake time) is the foundation of optimal sleep hygiene. It may become harder to exercise, or even to be exposed to natural light, both of which are important for establishing circadian rhythm. It may be easier to spend too much time in bed, or to nap excessively during the day. Most patients should adjust their schedule to the expected phase advance with aging, rather than try to stay up later than their peak sleepiness in the evening. All of these issues are more severe for those in any assisted living environment. Cognitive behavioral therapy for these issues may be particularly useful in the elderly (discussed elsewhere in this issue).

Medical Illness and Poor Sleep

Many illnesses, both medical and psychiatric, that are more common in the elderly, have profound effects on sleep.[10] Any disease associated with pain may lead to fragmented sleep. Cardiac and respiratory illnesses, including congestive heart failure, chronic obstructive pulmonary disease, and asthma, are commonly worse in sleep. Worsened breathing may be related to the recumbent position or by the respiratory drive reduction accompanying sleep. Hypoxemia and hypercapnia are slight at sleep onset, but are more noticeable in REM sleep. Chronic renal failure or anemia may cause or worsen symptoms of restless legs syndrome and periodic limb movements of sleep, leading to problems with sleep maintenance. Common medications may have changes on sleep architecture that are not always obvious. For example, beta-blockers are commonly associated with complaints of nightmares and increased dream recall, despite their effect of reducing REM sleep, because of increased awakenings. Sleep changes are more common with lipophilic beta-blockers.[11,12] Other conditions that commonly worsen sleep or worsen with sleep include arthritis, dementia, prostatic hypertrophy, depression, and anxiety.

EPIDEMIOLOGY OF SLEEP APNEA IN THE ELDERLY

Data regarding the prevalence of sleep apnea in the elderly are limited by inconsistent definitions. An apnea is a cessation of breathing lasting at least 10 seconds. Apneas

---

Box 1
Taking a sleep history

What time do you go to bed?

How long does it take to fall asleep?

Do you wake during the night (how many times)?

What time do you get out of bed in the morning?

Have you been observed to snore, gasp, choke, or stop breathing during your sleep?

Do you have trouble staying awake during the day?

---

may be obstructive (absent airflow with continued respiratory effort) or central (no effort). Hypopneas may be equally important in assessing breathing during sleep, but they have been defined by at least 2 separate conventions. In the 2012 standard of the American Academy of Sleep Medicine, a hypopnea is defined as a 30% or greater reduction in airflow accompanied by either an EEG arousal or a 3% oxygen desaturation.[13] The Centers for Medicare and Medicaid Services requires a 4% oxygen desaturation and does not accept an arousal. It may be difficult to distinguish obstructive from central hypopneas. The number of apneas per hour is the apnea index (AI). The number of apneas and hypopneas per hour is expressed as the apnea-

---

Box 2
Epworth sleepiness questionnaire

How likely are you to nod off or fall asleep in the following situations, in contrast to feeling just tired? This refers to your usual way of life in recent times. Even if you haven't done some of these things recently, try to work out how they would have affected you. It is important that you answer each question as best you can. Use the following scale to choose the most appropriate number for each situation:

Would never nod off: 0

Slight chance of nodding off: 1

Moderate chance of nodding off: 2

High chance of nodding off: 3

Sitting and reading :_____

Watching TV: _____

Sitting, inactive, in a public place (eg, in a meeting, theater, or dinner event): _____

As a passenger in a car for an hour or more without stopping for a break: _____

Lying down to rest when circumstances permit: _____

Sitting and talking to someone: _____

Sitting quietly after a meal without alcohol: _____

In a car, while stopped for a few minutes in traffic or at a light: _____

Add up your points to get your total score. A score of 10 or greater raises concern: you may need to get more sleep, improve your sleep practices, or seek medical attention to determine why you are sleepy.

Adapted from Johns MW. A new method for measuring daytime sleepiness: The Epworth Sleepiness Scale. Sleep 1991;14:540.

---

hypopnea index (AHI). Depending on the definition for hypopnea used, this number can vary greatly, and it can be difficult to compare some epidemiologic studies. Although there are drawbacks to using this measure to quantify sleep apnea, it has become standard in the literature.

Obstructive sleep apnea is far more common than central sleep apnea. The prevalence of obstructive sleep apnea clearly increases among older and less healthy individuals. In 1 study of patients referred for sleep evaluation, the prevalence of an AI of 10 or more was 10% among independent older adults, 21% on a medical ward, and 26% in nursing home residents.[14] In the Sleep Heart Health Study, a random sample of nearly 6000 subjects, with hypopnea defined by 4% desaturations, the prevalence of an AHI of 15 or greater increased by 24% for each 10-year age increment, with a possible leveling off after 60 years of age.[15] The prevalence of central sleep apnea was extremely low in this healthy population: 91% had less than 1 central event per hour. Central sleep apnea, which may be associated with periodic breathing (Cheyne-Stokes pattern), is commonly associated with cardiac or neurologic disease.

In general, the most common symptoms of sleep apnea are snoring and daytime sleepiness in both the elderly and younger adults.[16] However, cognitive deficits and nocturia may also be frequent presentations in the elderly. Sleep apnea is generally more common in men than women and is associated with obesity. However, the gender difference ends at about the time of menopause.[17] After the age of 50, gender becomes an unimportant variable, and the association with body mass index becomes insignificant.[18]

SUMMARY

Sleep changes with aging, but poor sleep is not necessarily universal and should be investigated. All evaluations should start with a sleep history (**Box 1**): at a minimum, patients (and their bed partner, if available) should be asked about usual bedtime, average time to fall asleep ("sleep latency"), number of awakenings, usual time to get out of bed in the morning, presence of daytime sleepiness, and observations of snoring. A sleep log may be informative, but is highly subjective and may be inaccurate, as it is difficult for anyone to accurately assess their own sleep. Patients must be questioned about medications, alcohol, and caffeine use. Given the number of illnesses that can cause or be associated with poor sleep, all patients need a general physical examination and basic laboratory tests. The complaint of excessive daytime sleepiness (EDS) is an important clue. Although this is very subjective, the Epworth questionnaire (**Box 2**) may be helpful. This questionnaire asks about the propensity to become sleepy on a scale of 0 to 3 under 8 conditions, so that a higher score indicates greater sleepiness.[19] A score greater than 10 is considered abnormal. The Epworth scale is not well validated in the elderly, however.

Patients whose complaints appear consistent with normal aging need not be further investigated. Daytime napping may be normal or even beneficial, but EDS should not be considered normal in the healthy elderly. Any patient who appears to be getting a reasonable amount of sleep (perhaps 7 hours) who has difficulty staying awake should have further evaluation. This further evaluation might include overnight polysomnography or home sleep testing. With the increased availability of polysomnography and improved accuracy and simplicity of home testing, sleep evaluation is becoming increasingly convenient. Some patients should be screened even in the absence of significant sleep symptoms: those with a history of stroke or transient ischemic attack have such a high prevalence of sleep-disordered breathing that testing should be routine. Patients with early dementia also might be routinely tested, as there is increased evidence that improvement or delaying of progression of symptoms with treatment for sleep apnea may occur, and symptoms may be difficult to assess.

CLINICS CARE POINTS

- Sleep changes with aging but complaints of poor sleep or daytime sleepiness should be investigated.
- Sleep disordered breathing may be a risk for stroke or dementia in the elders.

REFERENCES

1. United Nations, Department of Economic and Social Affairs, Population Division (2019). World Population Prospects 2019: Highlights (ST/ESA/SER.A/423).
2. Foley DJ, Monjan AA, Brown SL, et al. Sleep complaints among elderly persons: an epidemiologic study of three communities. Sleep 1995;18(6):425–32.
3. Foley DJ, Monjan A, Simonsick EM, et al. Incidence and remission of insomnia among elderly adults: an epidemiologic study of 6,800 persons over three years. Sleep 1999;22:S366–72.
4. Rechtshaffen A, Kales A. A manual of standardized terminology, techniques and scoring system for sleep stages of human subjects. Los Angeles (CA): UCLA Brain Information Service/Brain Research Institute; 1968.
5. Ohayon MM, Carskadon MA, Guilleminault C, et al. Meta-analysis of quantitative sleep parameters from childhood to old age in healthy individuals: developing normative sleep values across the human lifespan. Sleep 2004;27(7):1255–73.
6. Redline S, Kirchner HL, Quan SF, et al. The effects of age, sex, ethnicity, and sleep disordered breathing on sleep architecture. Arch Int Med 2004;164: 406–18.
7. Van Cauter E, Leproult R, Plat L. Age-related changes in slow wave sleep and REM sleep and relationship with growth hormone and cortisol levels in healthy men. JAMA 2000;284:861–8.
8. Dijk DJ, Groeger JA, Stanley N, et al. Age-related reduction in daytime sleep propensity and nocturnal slow wave sleep. Sleep 2010;33:211.
9. Duffy JF, Willson HJ, Wang W, et al. Healthy older adults better tolerate sleep deprivation than young adults. J Am Geriatr Soc 2009;57:1245–51.
10. Quan SF, Zee P. Evaluating the effects of medical disorders on sleep in the older patient. Geriatrics 2004;59:37.
11. Betts TA, Alford C. Beta-blockers and sleep: a controlled trial. Eur J Clin Pharmacol 1985;28(suppl):65–8.
12. Westerlund A. Central nervous system side-effects with hydrophilic and lipophilic beta-blockers. Eur J Clin Pharmacol 1985;28(suppl):73.
13. Berry RB, Budhiraja R, Gottlieb DJ, et al. Rules for scoring respiratory events in sleep: update of the 2007 AASM manual. J Clin Sleep Med 2012;8(5):597–619.
14. Ancoli-Israel S. Epidemiology of sleep disorders. Clin Geriatr Med 1989;5:347.
15. Young T, Shahar E, Nieto FJ, et al. Predictors of sleep-disordered breathing in community-dwelling adults. Arch Intern Med 2002;162(8):893–900.
16. Lévy P, Pépin JL, Malauzat D, et al. Is sleep apnea syndrome in the elderly a specific entity? Sleep 1996;19:S29.
17. Young T, Finn L, Austin D, et al. Menopausal status and sleep-disordered breathing in the Wisconsin Sleep Cohort Study. Am J Respir Crit Care Med 2003;167(9): 1181–5.

18. Tishler PV, Larkin EK, Schluchter MD, et al. Incidence of sleep-disordered breathing in an urban adult population: the relative importance of risk factors in the development of sleep-disordered breathing. JAMA 2003;289(17): 2230–7.
19. Johns MW. A new method for measuring daytime sleepiness: the Epworth Sleepiness Scale. Sleep 1991;14:540.

Insomnia
Behavioral Treatment in the Elderly

Matthew R. Ebben, PhD[a,b],*

KEYWORDS

- CBT-I • Elderly • Nonpharmacologic • Insomnia • Behavioral • Cognitive • Age

KEY POINTS

- Sleep issues in elderly individuals can often be attributed to increased mental and physical health problems associated with aging. Nonetheless, sleep drive decreases and fragmentation increases as we age.
- After the age of 20, circadian phase advances, causing many older patients to have an abnormally early sleep and wake time.
- Cognitive behavioral therapy for insomnia (CBT-I) is the preferred treatment approach for insomnia in all adults, including elderly individuals.
- Adding bright light therapy to CBT-I can help delay an advanced circadian phase.

INTRODUCTION

In this article, changes that occur in sleep with age, prevalence of insomnia, the most influential models explaining the development of insomnia, as well as nonpharmacologic treatment methods to improve poor-quality sleep are concisely reviewed within the context of older patients. In addition, other popular treatment techniques, such as sleep hygiene and melatonin use, are briefly mentioned.

AGE-RELATED CHANGES IN SLEEP ARCHITECTURE

Throughout the human life span, changes occur in the architecture, length, and quality of sleep.[1] During infancy and early childhood, we sleep more than any other point in postnatal life and spend a much larger percentage of time in both rapid-eye movement (REM) and slow-wave sleep (SWS).[2] Until the age of 60, total sleep time (TST), sleep efficiency, percentage of SWS, percentage of REM sleep, and REM latency all significantly decrease.[1] Wake after sleep onset, stage 1, and sleep latency are all increased

[a] Weill Medical College of Cornell University, Center for Sleep Medicine, 425 East 61st Street, 5th Floor, New York, NY 10065, USA; [b] Polysomnographic Technology Training Program, Kingsborough Community College (CUNY), 2001 Oriental Boulevard, Brooklyn, NY 11235, USA
* Weill Medical College of Cornell University, Center for Sleep Medicine, 425 East 61st Street, 5th Floor, New York, NY 10065.
E-mail address: mae2001@med.cornell.edu

in older compared with younger adults.[1,3] Many of the changes in sleep architecture, such as decreased REM and SWS, stabilize around the age of 60. Unfortunately, sleep efficiency continues to decline into old age.

INSOMNIA PREVALENCE

Insomnia is estimated to affect 6% to 15% of the population,[4] and is therefore one of the most prevalent health conditions worldwide. A large-scale epidemiologic study found that 23% to 34% of individuals older than 65 complained of symptoms consistent with insomnia, with more than 50% reporting difficulty sleeping (not reaching the level of insomnia).[5] Some have argued that changes in sleep architecture associated with aging are not indicative of reduced sleep need, but instead point toward reduced sleep ability, which is related to circadian rhythm alterations as well as psychiatric and health issues that tend to occur with age.[6] Moreover, once mental and medical health conditions are controlled for, the prevalence of insomnia in older adults is reduced and is similar to younger populations.[7] In addition, addressing mood and health conditions in elderly individuals often improves sleep quality. Nonetheless, insomnia remains a common complaint in elderly individuals and if not treated will decrease quality of life.

MODELS OF INSOMNIA
The 2-Process Model

Although not specifically a model of insomnia, the 2-Process model helps us to understand the factors that control alertness and sleep throughout the 24-hour day[8] and helps us to explain changes in sleep quality as we age. This model describes sleep propensity (homeostatic drive or process S) as a physiologic drive that builds in a monotonic fashion during periods of wakefulness. During sleep, this drive is relieved in the form of slow-wave activity (SWA) in the electroencephalogram. Periods of sleep deprivation result in a rebound of SWA during subsequent bouts of sleep, and naps during the day reduce SWA at night by reducing process S during the napping period.

Process C, the second part of the 2-Process model, describes the influence of circadian rhythms on sleep and alertness. This process is regulated by *zeitgebers* (German for time giver) that adapt various functions of the body to a 24-hour rhythm. In humans, light is a powerful zeitgeber.[9,10] Bright light exposure in the eyes of humans stimulates photosensitive retinal ganglion cells that transfer signals via the retinal hypothalamic pathway to the suprachiasmatic nucleus, which is the master clock of the body. The suprachiasmatic nucleus, through humoral and neuronal signals, regulates peripheral clocks throughout the body.[11]

As we age, changes in the circadian rhythm occur. In fact, Roenneberg and colleagues[12] proposed that the point of maximal delay and a subsequent shift to a more advanced circadian phase, which occurs at approximately 20 years of age, is an indication of a biological shift from adolescence to adulthood. Throughout adulthood and into old age, the circadian phase continues to advance.[12] Although the genetic properties of the circadian clock in cells throughout the body do not change in older adults, it has been hypothesized that a thermolabile factor in the blood serum of older individuals is responsible for a shortening of the circadian rhythms,[13] resulting in an advance of the sleep phase.

CHANGE IN CIRCADIAN PHASE WITH AGE

The advance in the circadian phase means that older individuals tend to both fall asleep and wake up earlier than younger individuals (**Fig. 1**).[14] In some cases, sleep

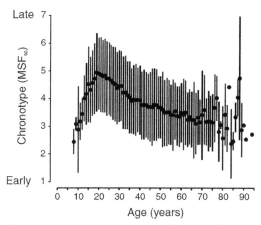

Fig. 1. Illustration of chronotype by age using the midpoint of sleep on free days derived from results on the Munich Chronotype Questionnaire. A higher value on the y-axis shows a more delayed circadian phase. (*From* Roenneberg T, Kuehnle T, Pramstaller PP, et al. A marker for the end of adolescence. *Curr Biol.* 2004;14(24):R1038-1039; with permission.)

can advance to the point of interfering with evening activities and can cause abnormally early morning wake-up times and may need to be treated. This is described in more detail later in this article.

The Spielman Model

The development of insomnia is complex, in part, because often the issues that led to the onset of disease are different from those that cause the difficulty sleeping to continue. Therefore, Spielman and colleagues[15] developed the 3-P (also known as the Spielman) model to help explain the change of insomnia over time from acute condition to chronic disease. The 3 P's in this model stand for predisposing, precipitating, and perpetuating factors.

Predisposing traits can be thought of as the underlying combination of both the personality makeup and the level of physiologic arousal of an individual and is relatively stable over time. The term hyperarousal is often used in the psychological literature to describe a specific predisposing trait that, if high, places a person at greater risk of developing insomnia. Folks with a high level of hyperarousal keep a consistently elevated level of vigilance. As a result, even small stressors can place these individuals at risk of acute difficulty sleeping.

Precipitating events are situations that create a high level of stress or change in lifestyle and can be either positive or negative in nature; for example, the death of someone close, changing jobs or careers, moving to a new home, or a serious conflict with someone, to name just a few instances. Nearly everyone encounters events that cause short-term difficulty sleeping. In most cases, once the stressful event dissipates, sleep returns to normal.

Perpetuating factors are behaviors that convert acute insomnia to a chronic condition. The single most damaging perpetuating activity to sleep is increasing time in bed (TIB). Often when people develop difficulty sleeping, they will increase TIB to help increase the chance that they will be able to recapture the lost sleep. However, if increased TIB is maintained for extended periods of time, it will almost certainly cause insomnia to become a chronic condition long after the original stressor has been resolved. Other perpetuating activities can include maladaptive behaviors, such as working on the computer, reading, watching TV, or eating in bed.

Neurocognitive Model

Perlis and colleagues[16] elaborated on the Spielman model by describing how repeated episodes of insomnia, which result in a combination of cortical, cognitive, and somatic arousal, result in a classically conditioned hyperaroused response to sleep-related stimuli. Once conditioned, hyperarousal becomes a perpetuating factor that persists long after precipitating events cease to play a role in elevating stress. This theory is evidenced by studies showing increased cortical arousal in people with insomnia.[17–20]

Attention-Intention-Effort Pathway

Another framework to help understand insomnia has been proposed by Colin Espie and colleagues.[21] This model is called the Attention-Intention-Effort pathway. This theory describes how difficulty sleeping is worsened or perpetuated by direct attention on an activity that is normally an automatic process. In other words, good sleepers do not think about the process of falling asleep and maintaining sleep. However, as sleep quality degrades, attention becomes focused on the process of sleeping, which in turn causes increased arousal and turns an acute insomnia into a chronic condition.

Two-Factor Model

Developed by Bonnet and Arand in the late 1990s,[22] the 2-factor model describes insomnia as involving 2 competing drives. One is the physiologic arousal level of the individual and the other is the sleep drive. Having a low sleep drive or an elevated level of arousal predisposes a person to insomnia. This model is based, in part, on studies that show, despite inadequate sleep, people with insomnia are less sleepy than those with normal sleep when given a multiple sleep latency test,[23] which is an objective test of daytime sleepiness. Moreover, when normal sleepers are experimentally driven to higher levels of anxiety, they tend to develop poor-quality sleep.[24] This model has good face validity because it is easy to relate to having trouble sleeping after a stressful day, even if one does not consider oneself to be an insomniac. The 2-Factor model explains this phenomenon through a brief increase in arousal level due to the stressful day, which acutely surpasses the level of sleep drive.

The 2-Factor model is simple to understand and describes 2 important targets of treatment. Therefore, it is useful to use this model to describe insomnia to patients, particularly when focusing on a treatment approach such as sleep restriction therapy (SRT; described in more detail later in this article), which is designed to increase sleep drive to overcome the arousal level of the individual with insomnia. Describing SRT in terms of the 2-Factor model helps patients to understand the theory behind reducing TIB to help increase sleep drive, and how a high sleep drive can overcome elevated levels of anxiety without focusing directly on the anxiety.

Nonpharmacologic Treatment Models for Insomnia

According to the American College of Physicians, cognitive behavioral therapy for insomnia (CBT-I) should be used as the first-line treatment for primary insomnia.[25] Although hypnotic medication can be useful for acute insomnia, CBT-I is the preferred long-term treatment choice for difficulty sleeping because it addresses the factors that perpetuate the problem. CBT-I is a multi-element therapy that includes stimulus control, cognitive therapy, relaxation-based treatment, and sleep restriction (**Table 1** below).

Table 1
The first recommendation listed is the current guideline[26]

Therapeutic Approach	Focus of Intervention	AASM Level of Recommendation
Multicomponent cognitive behavioral therapy	Using all the techniques listed below in combination.	[a]Standard[26] (+Strong[27])
Stimulus control	Conditioning the bed and bedroom to be associated with sleep	[a]Standard[26] (++Conditional[27])
Cognitive therapy	Restructuring maladaptive thought processes about sleep	[a]Standard[26] (+++No recommendation[27])
Relaxation-based treatment	Reducing tension	[a]Standard[26] (Conditional[27])
Sleep restriction	Increasing sleep drive to overcome level of arousal	[b]Guideline[26] (Conditional[27])
Mindfulness	Teaching nonjudgmental awareness to help reduce anxiety about sleep	N/A[26] (+++No recommendation[27])
Sleep hygiene	A collection of behaviors or actions that should either be avoided or adopted to improve sleep quality	+++No recommendation[26] (Conditional recommendation not to use[27])

The American Academy of Sleep Medicine's (AASM) level of recommendation in brackets shows the recently released (2021) recommendations.[27] +Strong: Indicates a treatment that will benefit most patients. ++Conditional: A recommended treatment that should be used based on clinical judgment. +++No recommendation: A treatment without adequate evidence of benefit. N/A: not assessed in review.
[a] Standard: This is a generally accepted patient-care strategy that reflects a high degree of clinical certainty.
[b] Legend: This is a patient-care strategy that reflects a moderate degree of clinical certainty.

More recently, mindfulness-based interventions also have been added to the armamentarium.

COGNITIVE BEHAVIORAL THERAPY FOR INSOMNIA TREATMENT MODALITY, FOCUS OF INTERVENTION, AND LEVEL OF AMERICAN ACADEMY OF SLEEP MEDICINE RECOMMENDATION
Stimulus Control Therapy

Originally developed by Bootzin[28] and based on operant conditioning, stimulus control therapy is the concept that pairing waking activities with the bed and bedroom prevents the conditioned association of the bed with sleep. For example, consistently pairing TV watching, reading, and/or eating in bed will result in the bed and bedroom being associated with activities related to wakefulness, whereas if the bed and bedroom are only used for sleep, it increases the likelihood that sleep will occur when getting into bed. Therefore, with repeated pairings, the bed becomes a discriminative stimulus to sleep onset. The goal of stimulus control treatment is to condition the bed and bedroom with sleep. To carry out this task, the following recommendations are made[29]:

1. Only get into bed when sleepy.
2. Get out of bed if unable to sleep (after 20 minutes).
3. Eliminate wake-promoting activities from the bed and bedroom.
4. Wake at the same time each morning.
5. Avoid napping.

Several studies have shown stimulus control to be an effective treatment for insomnia. Therefore, the American Academy of Sleep Medicine (AASM) considers this part of CBT-I to be a "standard" therapy, which is the Academy's highest recommendation.[26] As a result, elements of stimulus control are often used in the successful treatment of insomnia.

Cognitive Therapy

Cognitive therapy for insomnia focuses on irrational beliefs about sleep, unrealistic expectations, catastrophizing, and over valuing the need for sleep.[30] Those with insomnia can enter a negative thought loop where difficulty sleeping initiates a cascade of counterproductive thoughts about the insomnia. For example, while lying in bed not sleeping, one may begin looking at the clock to calculate how much sleep is possible before their required morning wake time. Feeling that the remaining sleep time is insufficient, even if they fell asleep at once, they may ruminate about being unable to perform at work, resulting in job loss, or they may worry about developing a catastrophic disease due to inadequate sleep. This downward spiral of thoughts decreases the likelihood that they will fall back to sleep and further worsens the insomnia.

Therefore, the focus of cognitive therapy is to break the cycle of negative thoughts and restructure thought processes to have more realistic expectations about sleep. To help control presleep rumination, the use of a worry list in conjunction with thought stopping may be helpful. A worry list (otherwise known as a Pennebaker writing task[31]) is a list constructed by the patient 1 to 2 hours before sleep. This list has all the issues the patient is worried about and how they intend to address these concerns the following day.[32] Issues that cannot be addressed will be deferred until the next day. Once the list has been written, the patient is instructed to avoid thinking about problems on the list. If they find themselves ruminating about an item on the worry list, they are advised to stop the thought at once and begin thinking about another topic. Of note, the empirical data on the benefit of this approach are mixed; Harvey and Ferral[33] found it to significantly improve sleep onset latency, but in a more recent study this finding was not replicated.[34]

One of the more fascinating cognitive interventions for insomnia is called paradoxic intention (this method is often listed separately from cognitive therapy, but is essentially a specific type of cognitive approach). This strategy requires the patient to avoid trying to sleep and instead remain in bed awake as long as possible. The patient is advised to avoid extreme or painful techniques to stay awake, and instead simply lie in bed calmly with their eyes closed. By reducing the anxiety associated with trying to sleep, paradoxic intention has been shown to reduce sleep latency and improve overall sleep quality.[35]

Relaxation-Based Treatments

Relaxation-based methods to help improve sleep quality have also been investigated. These techniques focus on tension as the source of the insomnia. One of the most common relaxation therapies that focuses on somatic tension is progressive muscle relaxation. To use this method, patients are instructed to begin at the head, and systematically tense then relax each muscle group until they have reached their toes. Although effective in some patient populations, progressive muscle relaxation has been shown to worsen insomnia in those who do not report somatic tension.[36]

When rumination occurs during sleep, and a worry list with thought stopping is ineffective, creative visualization can be helpful. This process involves having the patient create a story that they visualize during sleep. The story can involve anything the patient finds relaxing, but must follow a few simple rules:

1. The story cannot include any other people.
2. It must be as detailed as possible.
3. The plot needs to have a beginning, middle, and end.

Visualizing this story when awake at night allows the patient to replace anxiety-producing thoughts with more relaxing mentations. This can hasten sleep onset.

Sleep Restriction Therapy

SRT, developed by Art Spielman and colleagues,[37] reduces TIB to match average sleep time, to improve nighttime sleep quality. To carry out this task, a patient is instructed to complete a sleep log (**Fig. 2**) each morning upon awakening. On this log, bedtime, periods of sleep, and time out of bed are documented typically for a period of at least 2 weeks. Average nightly TST is calculated from this log, and the patient is then asked to limit TIB to the TST from the previous 2 weeks. Once sleep quality improves, if sleepiness remains, TIB is slowly increased until daytime alertness improves.

When the proper sleep period is chosen in SRT, the result is an increase in homeostatic sleep drive. Over time, this increases the likelihood of sleep occurring during the prescribed sleep period. Although considered a guideline treatment for insomnia (1 step lower than a standard treatment) by AASM,[26] many consider SRT to be one of the most effective elements of CBT-I,[38] if not the most effective part. The reason this aspect of CBT-I is so effective, is because when performed correctly, SRT includes principal elements of stimulus control and cognitive therapy and helps align circadian rhythms. This statement may be surprising to some, but let us consider practical elements of implementing SRT.

After having a patient complete sleep logs and selecting a new sleep-wake schedule, the patient is advised to maintain a limited TIB with a fixed sleep and

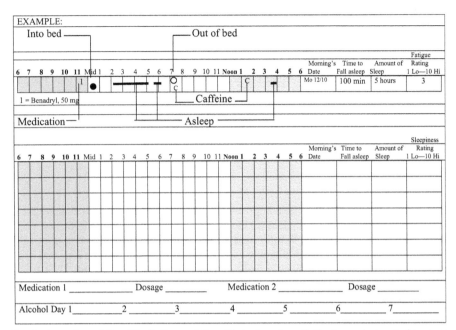

Fig. 2. A version of the City College of New York sleep log. Patients are instructed to complete this each morning. The black dot indicates the time the patient got into bed, and the black lines represent periods of sleep. The black circle shows time out of bed. The numeral before the black dot indicates when medications were taken (if any were taken before bedtime). Medications taken at other times of the day are listed below the chart. c indicates time of caffeine consumption. Daily alcohol consumption for each day is listed below medications. (*From* Ebben MR, Spielman AJ. Non-pharmacological treatments for insomnia. J Behav Med. 2009;32(3):244-254; with permission.)

wake time. Moreover, patients are asked to avoid napping. Therefore, 2 elements of stimulus control, avoiding napping and waking up at the same time each day, are part of the SRT instructions. In addition, keeping a fixed TIB helps to entrain circadian rhythms over time. The cognitive aspects of SRT are required to convince patients to follow the restricted schedule. Patients often complain about the risks of reducing TIB and the resulting sleep loss, and how this may negatively affect their long-term health and daytime functioning. This allows the practitioner an opportunity to discuss realistic expectations about sleep, and address catastrophizing and overvaluing the need for sleep.

Mindfulness-Based Interventions

Mindfulness is the primary focus of Buddhist psychology, which teaches patients nonjudgmental awareness. In the field of behavioral sleep medicine, mindfulness-based stress reduction (MBSR) has received growing attention in the literature.[39] The MBSR program teaches meditation, breathing techniques, and body scanning as tools of self-awareness and is often taught in a group setting. This technique can be helpful in patients who tend to catastrophize when unable to sleep. Teaching acceptance of the act of not sleeping can help to reduce anxiety during awakenings at night, or when having difficulty falling asleep. Often MBSR is combined with behavioral techniques such as SRT to improve efficacy.

Sleep Hygiene Education

The term sleep hygiene was originally coined by Peter Hauri[40] to describe a collection of behaviors that should be either avoided or adopted to improve sleep quality. Although these recommendations vary based on the source, they tend to have excellent face validity. As a result, over time they have become imprinted in the consciousness of the general public as the path to superior quality sleep. Unfortunately, sleep hygiene has not been consistently shown to be an effective standalone therapy for insomnia and is therefore not recognized by AASM as a validated treatment technique.[26] Regrettably, many people with insomnia conflate sleep hygiene with effective CBT-I methods. Consequently, after rigidly adhering to sleep hygiene and seeing no appreciable benefit, some individuals become disenchanted with nonpharmacologic interventions for insomnia before even trying them.

Considerations for Treating Insomnia in Older Populations

In older adults, often the onset of insomnia is more gradual in nature. This is due to lifestyle changes associated with retirement (or reduced work hours) and a decrease in social and/or physical activities. Frequently reduced daytime activities and a more flexible schedule result in increased TIB. For those who kept a chronic partial sleep-deprived state during their working years, the increased TIB may initially result in increased TST and feeling more alert during the day. However, once their sleep debt has been discharged, the added TIB results in a fragmentation of sleep over the longer period in bed. When insomnia develops in this fashion, the precipitating event is the change in lifestyle and not an acute increase in stress due to a temporary event. As a result, when conceptualized in the framework of the 3-P model, both the precipitating and perpetuating factors are one and the same.

There is also evidence that the homeostatic sleep drive changes with age. Studies have shown that when compared with younger individuals, homeostatic drive in response to sleep deprivation is reduced in elderly individuals, particularly in the frontal regions of the brain.[41] Moreover, the discharge of SWA becomes less pronounced with age,[3] suggesting that older patients have different treatment needs than younger individuals. Meta-analytic studies have shown CBT-I to be effective in elderly individuals.[42,43] In addition, when investigated alone, SRT has been shown to be an effective treatment method in older patients, and may be more effective than a purely cognitive approach.[43] This suggests that older patients may benefit more from treatment techniques that strengthen the homeostatic drive.

As mentioned in the introduction, beginning in the late teens to early 20s, circadian rhythms shift from a more delayed to a more advanced phase.[12] In some, the advance is so pronounced that it interferes with social activities in the evening and can result in persistent early morning awakenings. This condition is referred to as advanced sleep phase syndrome, and is more common in older patients.[44] This may be due to a combination of changes in the eye that occur with age, which can lead to less light intake,[45] and a reduction in both period length and amplitude of the circadian rhythm.[46] Systematic exposure to bright light at the proper circadian time, a treatment approach called bright light therapy, can help treat this condition.[47] A recent study in institutionalized elderly patients found that bright light exposure in the evening significantly improved sleep quality, cognitive function, and delayed circadian rhythms.[48]

Using Melatonin in Elderly Patients

One of the most common over-the-counter sleep aids is melatonin. Often, this medication is taken at bedtime in the hopes that it will hasten the onset of sleep, or, particularly in elderly individuals, delay terminal awakenings in the morning. However, the use of melatonin in aged patients presents unique problems. To understand why melatonin is problematic in older patients, we need to appreciate the phase response curve of melatonin in humans. A phase response curve is a term used in the field of circadian rhythm research to describe the change in circadian phase caused by a *zeitgeber*. We have already described the importance of bright light exposure in humans, which is a powerful *zeitgeber*.[9,10] However, exogenous melatonin can also act as a phase shifting agent in humans.[49] Whereas bright light exposure in the evening causes a delay of circadian rhythms, taking melatonin in the evening causes an advance.[50] Therefore, taking melatonin at bedtime can worsen early morning awakenings, which is a frequent problem in elderly patients, because of a tendency of the circadian rhythm to advance with age.[12,14] Therefore, melatonin should be used with caution in older patients and not for early morning awakenings.

SUMMARY

As we age, homeostatic sleep drive becomes weaker, and dissipates at a slower rate over the course of the night. Stage 1 sleep is increased as is sleep latency and wake after sleep onset, resulting in lighter more fragmented sleep. In addition, lifestyle changes that often result in a more flexible daytime schedule due to retirement, either resulting in or combined with circadian phase advances cause a significant decrease in overall sleep quality. CBT-I has been shown to improve insomnia in elderly individuals and should be used to blunt the effects of aging on sleep, particularly elements of therapy that focus on increasing homeostatic sleep drive, such as SRT. In addition, bright light therapy, when used in conjunction with CBT-I can help delay the circadian phase, which helps entrain sleep to occur at a more socially acceptable time.

CLINICS CARE POINTS

- Successful treatment of insomnia should focus on increasing sleep drive to overcome hyperarousal and recondition the patient to sleep in their bedroom environment.
- Using Sleep Restriction Therapy in conjunction with Stimulus Control and Cognitive Therapy is an effective way to increase sleep drive and recondition the patient to associate the bed with sleep.
- It is important to understand the circadian phase of each patient to ensure that the correct treatment approach is utilized.

REFERENCES

1. Ohayon MM, Carskadon MA, Guilleminault C, et al. Meta-analysis of quantitative sleep parameters from childhood to old age in healthy individuals: developing normative sleep values across the human lifespan. Sleep 2004;27(7):1255–73.
2. Roffwarg HP, Muzio JN, Dement WC. Ontogenetic development of the human sleep-dream cycle. Science 1966;152(3722):604–19.
3. Landolt HP, Borbély AA. Age-dependent changes in sleep EEG topography. Clin Neurophysiol 2001;112(2):369–77.
4. Ohayon MM. [Prevalence and comorbidity of sleep disorders in general population]. Rev Prat 2007;57(14):1521–8.
5. Foley DJ, Monjan AA, Brown SL, et al. Sleep complaints among elderly persons: an epidemiologic study of three communities. Sleep 1995;18(6):425–32.

6. Ancoli-Israel S, Alessi C. Sleep and aging. Am J Geriatr Psychiatry 2005;13(5): 341–3.
7. Foley DJ, Monjan A, Simonsick EM, et al. Incidence and remission of insomnia among elderly adults: an epidemiologic study of 6,800 persons over three years. Sleep 1999;22(Suppl 2):S366–72.
8. Borbely AA. A two process model of sleep regulation. Hum Neurobiol 1982;1(3): 195–204.
9. Wever RtA. The circadian system of man : results of experiments under temporal isolation. New York: Springer-Verlag; 1979.
10. Lewy AJ. Effects of light on human melatonin production and the human circadian system. Prog Neuropsychopharmacol Biol Psychiatry 1983;7(4–6):551–6.
11. Gachon F, Nagoshi E, Brown SA, et al. The mammalian circadian timing system: from gene expression to physiology. Chromosoma 2004;113(3):103–12.
12. Roenneberg T, Kuehnle T, Pramstaller PP, et al. A marker for the end of adolescence. Curr Biol 2004;14(24):R1038–9.
13. Pagani L, Schmitt K, Meier F, et al. Serum factors in older individuals change cellular clock properties. Proc Natl Acad Sci U S A 2011;108(17):7218–23.
14. Duffy JF, Dijk DJ, Klerman EB, et al. Later endogenous circadian temperature nadir relative to an earlier wake time in older people. Am J Physiol 1998;275(5 Pt 2):R1478–87.
15. Spielman AJ, Caruso LS, Glovinsky PB. A behavioral perspective on insomnia treatment. Psychiatr Clin North Am 1987;10(4):541–53.
16. Perlis ML, Giles DE, Mendelson WB, et al. Psychophysiological insomnia: the behavioural model and a neurocognitive perspective. J Sleep Res 1997;6(3): 179–88.
17. Freedman RR. EEG power spectra in sleep-onset insomnia. Electroencephalogr Clin Neurophysiol 1986;63(5):408–13.
18. Merica H, Blois R, Gaillard JM. Spectral characteristics of sleep EEG in chronic insomnia. Eur J Neurosci 1998;10(5):1826–34.
19. Perlis ML, Smith MT, Andrews PJ, et al. Beta/Gamma EEG activity in patients with primary and secondary insomnia and good sleeper controls. Sleep 2001;24(1): 110–7.
20. Perlis ML, Kehr EL, Smith MT, et al. Temporal and stagewise distribution of high frequency EEG activity in patients with primary and secondary insomnia and in good sleeper controls. J Sleep Res 2001;10(2):93–104.
21. Espie CA, Broomfield NM, MacMahon KM, et al. The attention-intention-effort pathway in the development of psychophysiologic insomnia: a theoretical review. Sleep Med Rev 2006;10(4):215–45.
22. Bonnet MH, Arand DL. Hyperarousal and insomnia. Sleep Med Rev 1997;1(2): 97–108.
23. Stepanski E, Zorick F, Roehrs T, et al. Daytime alertness in patients with chronic insomnia compared with asymptomatic control subjects. Sleep 1988;11(1):54–60.
24. Bonnet MH, Arand DL. Caffeine use as a model of acute and chronic insomnia. Sleep 1992;15(6):526–36.
25. Qaseem A, Kansagara D, Forciea MA, et al. Clinical Guidelines Committee of the American College of P. Management of chronic insomnia disorder in adults: a clinical practice guideline from the American College of Physicians. Ann Intern Med 2016;165(2):125–33.
26. Morgenthaler T, Kramer M, Alessi C, et al. Practice parameters for the psychological and behavioral treatment of insomnia: an update. An american academy of sleep medicine report. Sleep 2006;29(11):1415–9.

27. Edinger JD, Arnedt JT, Bertisch SM, et al. Behavioral and psychological treatments for chronic insomnia disorder in adults: an American Academy of Sleep Medicine clinical practice guideline. J Clin Sleep Med. 2021;17(2):255–62.

28. Bootzin RR. Stimulus control treatment for insomnia. Proc Am Psychol Assoc 1972;7:395–6.

29. Bootzin R, Epstein D, Wood JM. Critical issues in psychiatry: case studies in insomnia. In: Hauri P, editor. Stimulus control instructions. New York: Plenum Medical Book; 1991. p. 19–28.

30. Morin CM. Insomnia: psychological assessment and management. New York: Guilford Press; 1993.

31. Pennebaker JW, Beall SK. Confronting a traumatic event: toward an understanding of inhibition and disease. J abnormal Psychol 1986;95(3):274–81.

32. Lindsay WR, Gamsu CV, McLaughlin E, et al. A controlled trial of treatments for generalized anxiety. Br J Clin Psychol 1987;26(Pt 1):3–15.

33. Harvey AG, Farrell C. The efficacy of a Pennebaker-like writing intervention for poor sleepers. Behav Sleep Med 2003;1(2):115–24.

34. Mooney P, Espie CA, Broomfield NM. An experimental assessment of a Pennebaker writing intervention in primary insomnia. Behav Sleep Med 2009;7(2): 99–105.

35. Asher L, Turner R. Paradoxical intention and insomnia: an experimental investigation. Behav Res Ther 1979;17:408–11.

36. Hauri PJ, Percy L, Hellekson C, et al. The treatment of psychophysiologic insomnia with biofeedback: a replication study. Biofeedback Self Regul 1982; 7(2):223–35.

37. Spielman AJ, Saskin P, Thorpy MJ. Treatment of chronic insomnia by restriction of time in bed. Sleep 1987;10(1):45–56.

38. Perlis M, Shaw PJ, Cano G, et al. Chapter 78 - models of insomnia. 5th edition. Elsevier Inc; 2011.

39. Ong J, Sholtes D. A mindfulness-based approach to the treatment of insomnia. J Clin Psychol 2010;66(11):1175–84.

40. Hauri P. Critical issues in psychiatry: case studies in insomnia. In: Hauri P, editor. Sleep hygiene, relaxation therapy, and cognitive interventions. New York: Plenum Medical Book; 1991. p. 65–84.

41. Münch M, Knoblauch V, Blatter K, et al. The frontal predominance in human EEG delta activity after sleep loss decreases with age. Eur J Neurosci 2004;20(5): 1402–10.

42. Irwin MR, Cole JC, Nicassio PM. Comparative meta-analysis of behavioral interventions for insomnia and their efficacy in middle-aged adults and in older adults 55+ years of age. Health Psychol 2006;25(1):3–14.

43. McCurry SM, Logsdon RG, Teri L, et al. Evidence-based psychological treatments for insomnia in older adults. Psychol Aging 2007;22(1):18–27.

44. Ando K, Kripke DF, Ancoli-Israel S. Delayed and advanced sleep phase symptoms. Isr J Psychiatry Relat Sci 2002;39(1):11–8.

45. Zhou QP, Jung L, Richards KC. The management of sleep and circadian disturbance in patients with dementia. Curr Neurol Neurosci Rep 2012;12(2):193–204.

46. Weitzman ED, Moline ML, Czeisler CA, et al. Chronobiology of aging: temperature, sleep-wake rhythms and entrainment. Neurobiol Aging 1982;3(4):299–309.

47. Lewy AJ, Sack RA, Singer CL. Assessment and treatment of chronobiologic disorders using plasma melatonin levels and bright light exposure: the clock-gate model and the phase response curve. Psychopharmacol Bull 1984;20(3):561–5.

48. Rubiño JA, Gamundí A, Akaarir M, et al. Bright light therapy and circadian cycles in institutionalized elders. Front Neurosci 2020;14:359.
49. Arendt J, Bojkowski C, Folkard S, et al. Some effects of melatonin and the control of its secretion in humans. Ciba Found Symp 1985;117:266–83.
50. Burgess HJ, Revell VL, Eastman CI. A three pulse phase response curve to three milligrams of melatonin in humans. J Physiol 2008;586(2):639–47.

Insomnia
Pharmacologic Treatment

Becky X. Lou, MD[a],*, Margarita Oks, MD[b]

KEYWORDS

- Insomnia • Pharmacology • Geriatrics • Elderly • Adverse effects

KEY POINTS

- Secondary causes of insomnia, such as adverse effects of medications and medical conditions, should be reconciled before prescribing hypnotics.
- A dual approach with cognitive behavioral therapy and short-term hypnotics has been found to be effective in the treatment of insomnia.
- Prescribing hypnotics should be done with extreme caution particularly in the elderly.
- The risks of adverse effects and drug interactions should be thoroughly reviewed and weighed against the benefits of prescribing hypnotics.
- Newer hypnotics agents such as dual orexin receptor antagonists have more tolerable adverse effects.

INTRODUCTION

Insomnia has weighed heavily on the minds of many, including Shakespeare, who laments "O sleep, O gentle sleep, Nature's soft nurse, how have I frightened thee?"[1] Although insomnia is a common complaint among patients, The International Classification of Sleep Disorders—Third Edition recognizes insomnia with the following criteria: (1) patients having difficulty initiating or maintaining sleep despite (2) adequate circumstances and opportunity to sleep, which ultimately (3) affects their ability to function during the day.[2]

The diagnosis of insomnia continues to be highly prevalent worldwide. In the United States, insomnia affects nearly one-half of the elderly population.[3] Insomnia alone is associated with greater use of health services (ie, hospitalization, readmission, and emergency room visits).[4] And although the mainstay of insomnia lies in stimulus control and cognitive behavioral therapy, the addition of a hypnotic may still be required to achieve better quality sleep for the patient. The challenge with many pharmacologic

[a] Northwell Sleep Medicine Fellowship, Division of Pulmonary, Critical Care and Sleep Medicine, Department of Medicine, Donald and Barbara Zucker School of Medicine-Northwell, 410 Lakeville Road, Suite 107, New Hyde Park, NY 11042, USA; [b] Division of Pulmonary, Critical Care and Sleep Medicine, Department of Medicine, Donald and Barbara Zucker School of Medicine-Northwell, 100 East 77 Street, New York, NY 10075, USA
* Corresponding author.
E-mail address: Blou@northwell.edu

Clin Geriatr Med 37 (2021) 401–415
https://doi.org/10.1016/j.cger.2021.04.003
0749-0690/21/© 2021 Elsevier Inc. All rights reserved.

agents in treating elderly patients lies in a careful balance between efficacy and avoidance of detrimental adverse effects, as well as drug interactions.

PHYSIOLOGY OF WAKE AND SLEEP

Although the physiology of chronic insomnia is complex, neurotransmitters and their respective receptors have been identified as part of alerting systems within the brain making them potential pharmacologic targets. Although the generation of sleep and its neural networks are multifaceted, neurotransmitters can be generalized into either sleep or wake promoting.

Sensory and somatic inputs provide information from the medulla, midbrain, and posterior hypothalamus projecting to the thalamus, hypothalamus, basal forebrain, and cortex—ultimately creating the ascending reticular formation. This wake-promoting system depends on several neurotransmitters, including acetylcholine, norepinephrine, histamine, dopamine, and serotonin. Orexin, also known as hypocretin, which is secreted from the lateral hypothalamus, helps to regulate these arousal pathways, and its absence is key in the pathogenesis of narcolepsy which is a disease characterized by hypersomnolence.[5] Sleep is promoted by the removal of excitatory inputs from these neurotransmitters, and thus many inhibitory pharmacologic agents with these neurotransmitters in mind have been created to promote sleep.

Sleep-promoting systems depend on gamma-aminobutyric acid (GABA), the primary inhibitory neurotransmitter within the central nervous system. During the switch from wake to sleep, there is an increase in GABA activity to promote the inhibition of these thalamocortical pathways. GABA receptors have 5 subunits (2 ß, 2 α, and 1 γ subunits) with a central chloride ion channel pore. Several of these subunits serve as binding sites for benzodiazepines as well as nonbenzodiazepine "Z drugs" (including zolpidem, zaleplon, and zopiclone) and thus promote sleep.[6]

Last, melatonin, which is a hormone secreted from the pineal gland, helps to maintain and synchronize circadian rhythm. There are 2 receptor targets: MT1, which helps to attenuate arousal, and MT2, which is involved in the circadian rhythm cycles.[7] There are several medications that target the melatonin pathway for circadian rhythm problems as well as for sleep onset not related to circadian disturbance.

MEDICATIONS

Although cognitive behavioral therapy for insomnia, sleep restriction, and stimulus control should be used as much as possible in the treatment of insomnia, often the addition of hypnotics is required to achieve the desired quality of sleep for patients. Combination therapy with a hypnotic and cognitive behavioral therapy for insomnia is more effective than hypnotics or behavioral therapy alone.[8] Hypnotics should be tapered within 8 weeks, ideally.

Each patient's medical history and their medications, particularly in elderly patients who are prone to polypharmacy, should be carefully checked for adverse effects and interactions possible drug interactions with hypnotics. Clinicians should be mindful of wake-promoting agents that the patient may already be taking. Medications that can induce insomnia include selective serotonin reuptake inhibitors, serotonin and norepinephrine reuptake inhibitors, dopaminergic agents used for treating Parkinsonism as well as dementia, corticosteroids, and many cardiovascular agents, such as beta-blockers, calcium channel blockers, and statins[9] (**Table 1**). Underlying comorbidities should also be examined carefully, because insomnia can be caused by anxiety, depression, heart disease, dementia, or underlying sleep-disordered breathing.[10] Addressing these underlying conditions can help to resolve difficulty sleeping.

Table 1
Insomnia-inducing medications

Medication Type	Examples
Alpha-blockers	Doxazosin, prazosin, tamsulosin
Beta-blocker	Carvedilol, metoprolol, propranolol
Corticosteroids	Prednisone, dexamethasone, methylprednisolone
Calcium channel Blocker	Diltiazem, verapamil
Diuretics	Furosemide, bumetanide
Statins	Atorvastatin, rosuvastatin, simvastatin
Selective serotonin reuptake inhibitors	Fluoxetine, paroxetine, sertraline, citalopram, escitalopram
Serotonin and norepinephrine reuptake inhibitors	Bupropion (Wellbutrin), venlafaxine, duloxetine
Decongestants	Pseudoephedrine
Cholinesterase inhibitors	Donepezil, rivastigmine

The search for an ideal medication to combat insomnia has been ongoing. Before regimented clinical research and regulations, opioids, herbal supplements, and alcohol were commonly used to allay sleepless nights. In the early 1900s, barbiturates became the drug of choice to treat both sleep disturbances as well as epilepsy, but have fallen out of favor due to adverse effects and overdose potential.[11] Benzodiazepines were approved by the US Food and Drug Administration (FDA) in the 1960s and were rapidly incorporated by clinicians into patients' nighttime routines. However, the addictive properties of benzodiazepines along with fatal withdrawal symptoms also made them unfavorable for nightly use. In 1992, nonbenzodiazepines (eg, zolpidem) were approved by the FDA and have since continued to be the most prescribed hypnotic agents.[12] As research continues into the physiology of sleep, many sleep-promoting targets have been discovered, leading to many new, promising categories of drugs.

The American Academy of Sleep Medicine recently released a clinical guideline with recommendations on choosing pharmacologic agents for patients.[13,14] Several characteristics of these medications should be kept in mind, particularly the action onset, half-life duration, and potency of the drug. The pharmacodynamics of these drugs can be affected by age, and the geriatric population may have a more sensitive response to central nervous system drugs.[15] In general, many of these drugs are metabolized in the liver by the enzyme CYP3A4, so they should be used with extreme caution in patients with hepatic impairment or medications that may induce or inhibit CYP3A4. In addition, prescribers should be aware of any sleep-disordered breathing and lung disease, because some hypnotics can also decrease respiratory drive. The American Geriatric Society's Beer Criteria is another resource that has compiled potentially harmful, inappropriate medications for the elderly,[16] and can also be helpful in choosing the best hypnotic.

The various classes of pharmacologic agents are outlined, including benzodiazepines, "Z" drugs, antihistamines, dual orexin receptor antagonists, and melatonin agonists as well as a brief discussion on nonprescription hypnotic agents (**Table 2**). Antidepressants particularly tricyclics like amitriptyline are not recommended given their anticholinergic effects. Sedating antipsychotics such as quetiapine and olanzapine have not been well-studied in the context of insomnia.

Table 2
Hypnotic Dosing in the Geriatric Patient

Medication Category	Agents	Dose	Half-Life (h)	Metabolism	Peak Onset (h)	Major Adverse Effects
Benzodiazepine	Temazepam	7.5 mg Max: 30 mg	9–12	CYP3A4 (liver)	0.75–1.5	Increased risk of falls and injury Respiratory depression Cognitive dysfunction, ?dementia Tolerance/dependence, withdrawal Rebound anxiety, sleepiness in morning
	Triazolam	0.125 mg Max: 0.25 mg	1.5–5.5		0.75–2	
Z drugs	Eszopiclone	1 mg Max: 3 mg	9	CYP3A4 (liver)	1	NREM parasomnias including somnambulism and sleep-related eating disorder Psychomotor/cognitive impairment Increased risk of falls, injury ?Mortality
	Zolpidem	Ambien 5 mg Max: 10 mg Ambien CR 6.25 mg Max: 12.5 mg Edluar 5 mg Max: 10 mg Intermezzo 1.75 mg Max: 3.5 mg Zolpimist 5 mg Max: 10 mg	2.5 2.8 1.4–6.7 0.9		0.75–1.6	
	Zaleplon	5 mg Max: 10 mg	1	Aldehyde oxidase (liver)	1	
Antihistamine	Diphenhydramine	25 mg Max: 50 mg	3.4–9.2	CYP450 (liver)	1–4	Anticholinergic (diphenhydramine) Grogginess (diphenhydramine)
	Doxepin	3 mg Max: 6 mg	6–8	CYP2D6 (liver)	3.5	

Dual orexin receptor antagonists	Suvorexant	5 mg Max 20 mg	12	CYP3A4 (liver)	0.5–6	Dizziness
	Lemborexant	5 mg Max: 10 mg	17–19		1–3	?Increased risk of falls Contraindicated for narcolepsy
Melatonin	Melatonin	1 mg Max: 5 mg	1	CYP1A2 (liver)	1	Grogginess, nightmares, irritability, memory impairment (melatonin)
	Ramelteon	8 mg	1–2.5	CYP1A2 (liver)	0.5–1.5	Slight increase in fall risk
Antidepressant	Trazodone	12.5 mg Max: 50 mg	7–10	CYP3A4 (liver)	1–2	Prolonged QT, ventricular tachycardia, memory/cognitive impairment

Abbreviation: Max, maximum.

In general, hypnotic medications should be started at their lowest dose with a careful and slow monitored titration. Risks and benefits of hypnotic use should be discussed with patients so that their treatment can be approached as a shared decision. Close follow-up is necessary to monitor symptoms and their improvement.

Pharmacologic Agents

Benzodiazepine receptor agonists

Benzodiazepines have active binding sites within the GABA$_A$ receptor at the interface of the α and γ subunits (ie, "benzodiazepine site"). They act as modulators to GABA$_A$ receptors and help to promote sleep, mitigate anxiety, and act as an anticonvulsant. These agents are metabolized by CYP3A4 within the liver. Benzodiazepines have been approved for the treatment of insomnia. A variety of benzodiazepines are available for use, but more favorable results in regard to insomnia can be achieved by those with shorter half-lives. The American Academy of Sleep Medicine recommends the usage of short-acting agents, namely, temazepam and triazolam.[14]

Temazepam (Restoril). The most commonly used benzodiazepine is temazepam, which has a half-life of 9 to 12 hours and achieves significant blood levels in 30 minutes. The typical starting dose of temazepam is 15 mg at bedtime though for elderly patients it is recommended to start at 7.5 mg with maximum dosage of 30 mg at bedtime. Several randomized controlled trials showed a decrease in sleep latency and improvement in total sleep time with clinical significance.[17]

Triazolam (Halcion). Triazolam is another short-acting benzodiazepine with a half-life elimination of 1.5 to 5.5 hours and an onset of action within 15 to 30 minutes. The starting dose is 0.125 mg and can be increased to 0.250 mg at bedtime. There was a small decrease in mean sleep latency compared with placebo, but in a study within a geriatric population, triazolam showed a significant decrease in sleep onset time,[18] increased total sleep time, increased sleep efficiency, and decreased total wake time in the first three-quarters of the night.[19,20]

Adverse effects. Serious adverse effects and tolerance are major disadvantages of benzodiazepines, particularly in the elderly. The immediate adverse effects of benzodiazepines include dizziness, lethargy, dry mouth, headaches, an increased risk of falls resulting in devastating fractures, motor vehicle accidents, and memory impairment. There is also a risk of respiratory depression with escalating doses, and they should be used with caution in patients with sleep-disordered breathing and lung disease. Additionally, prolonged use could contribute to short-term and long-term cognitive dysfunction,[21] and there may also be an association with dementia.[22] Although short-acting benzodiazepines help to mitigate potential aftereffects, there remains a risk of rebound daytime anxiety or sleepiness the morning after use.

Tolerance, which is defined as decreased effectiveness with the same dose, has been well-documented, particularly in longer acting benzodiazepines, and can often persist for months to years after abstaining from the drug.[23] Slowly titrating off a benzodiazepine is also challenging, because rapid withdrawal symptoms can be potentially fatal. When titrating benzodiazepines, prescribers should follow the patient closely with extreme caution, observing for signs of withdrawal, including tremors, diaphoresis, palpitations, nausea, psychotic reactions, and seizures.[24]

Interestingly, a recent study examined the effects of withdrawing chronic temazepam and Z drugs (eg, zopiclone and zolpidem) in older adults. Although in the short term patients experienced rebound insomnia after each tapering dose, 6 months after the cessation of hypnotics, patients experienced less sleep disturbance, as well as improved daytime fatigue and quality of. The study also found that there was an improvement in muscle strength and balance in these patients.[25] These findings would favor the short-term use of benzodiazepines and Z drugs in the treatment of insomnia. Risks and benefits of benzodiazpine should be weighed for each individual patient.

Nonbenzodiazepine (Z drugs)

Nonbenzodiazepines, or Z drugs, are among the most commonly prescribed class of hypnotic medications. Like benzodiazepines, Z drugs such as zolpidem, zaleplon, and eszopiclone, target the $GABA_A$ receptors, although they have a selective affinity to particular subunits. These agents are also metabolized by CYP3A4 within the liver and should be used with caution in patients with hepatic dysfunction.

Eszopiclone (Lunesta). The longest acting of the Z drugs is eszopiclone and has a half-life of 9 hours in elderly patients with peak plasma levels achieved about 1 hour after administration. Eszopiclone targets the $GABA_A$ receptor's α1, 2, 3, and 5 subunits. A recent metanalysis that reviewed randomized control trials comparing various hypnotics showed that eszopiclone increases sleep duration compared with placebo objectively (28.6 minutes) and subjectively (25.08 minutes), as well as decrease subjective wake after sleep onset time and sleep efficiency when compared with placebo.[26] The typical starting dosage for eszopiclone is 1 mg at bedtime with maximum dose of 3 mg. However, in the geriatric population, maximum dosage of 3 mg may cause drowsiness and impairment during the day.

Zolpidem (Ambien, Intermezzo, Edluar, and Zolpimist). Zolpidem binds with high affinity to the α1 and α5 subunits on $GABA_A$ receptors. There are several different formulations with an intermediate half-life. The therapeutic onset for zolpidem is about 30 minutes. The most common is the immediate release zolpidem (Ambien), which has a half-life of 2.5 hours. The starting dose of the immediate release zolpidem is 5 mg and should not exceed 10 mg. There is also an extended-release zolpidem (Ambien CR), which has a half-life of 2.8 hours. The starting dosage is of 6.25 mg and should not exceed 12.5 mg. Sublingual (Edular, Sublinox, and Intermezzo) and nasal (Zolpimist) formulations also exist and have a half-life of 1.4 to 6.7 hours and 0.9 hours, respectively. These formulations come in both 5 mg and 10 mg, except Intermezzo which comes in 1.75 mg and 3.5 mg dosages. Like zolpidem, the starting dose should be 5 mg with a maximum dose of 10 mg.

Several randomized controlled trials have shown that zolpidem improves sleep by decreasing sleep latency, decreasing nocturnal awakenings, and improving sleep duration when compared with placebo.[27] However, many of these studies were limited by a study period of only 4 weeks. Therefore, the long-term effects of these medications have not been fully investigated and are felt to outweigh the benefits. All formulations of zolpidem can be used for sleep-onset insomnia, except for Intermezzo, which is recommended by the FDA for sleep-maintenance insomnia.

Zaleplon (Sonata). Zaleplon targets the $GABA_A$ receptor at its α1-3, β2, and γ2 subunits. It has a half-life of 1 hour with a rapid onset of action. It is also eliminated by the liver though primarily via aldehyde oxidase. The starting dose of zaleplon is 5 mg and can be increased to 10 mg. Zaleplon seems to be the most effective in decreasing sleep-onset latency when compared with controls both objectively and subjectively.[26] Because of its short half-life, it does not typically result in next-day effects and has been approved by the FDA for both sleep onset and maintenance insomnia.

Adverse effects. Common adverse effects of Z drugs include headaches, dizziness, nausea, and myalgias. Many studies have investigated potential adverse effects, particularly with regard to cognitive impairment and parasomnias, as well as the potential for falls and injury in the elderly. With Z drugs given at higher doses or if using extended-release formulas, residual effects of the hypnotic can be sustained into the next day, causing psychomotor and cognitive impairment. A systematic review and metanalysis found that there was a statistically significant increase in the risk for fractures, falls, and injuries using Z drugs, which can be particularly devastating to the geriatric population.[28] Another reported adverse effect is parasomnias, including sleep-related eating disorder, sleep driving, and somnambulism.[29] A retrospective analysis of the FDA's Adverse Event Reporting System over 16 years highlighted that there have been fatal cases owing to complex sleep behaviors.[30] Dependency, like with benzodiazepines, is also a potential risk and is about twice as common in those with a history of psychiatric diagnosis.[31] However, the relative incidences compared with benzodiazepines are lower.[32]

Of note, there has been a controversial association between hypnotic use and mortality, particularly those who used zolpidem.[33] Although some observational studies showed no link between hypnotic use and mortality, other studies showed a significant increase in mortality among elderly patients who use hypnotics. However, many of these studies seemed to be flawed owing to significant confounding factors, such as comorbidities, socioeconomic classes, sleep disorders, and underlying psychiatric disease. When these confounders were controlled, the risk of mortality was not associated with hypnotic use.[34] In addition, no study has investigated the cumulative effects or long-term effects of hypnotics in the elderly population. Nevertheless, given this potential link, this class of hypnotics should be used with great caution in the elderly, especially in those with multiple comorbidities, until further studies can clarify this potentially causal relationship.

Antihistamines

Histamine is not only involved in immune responses and regulating gastric release, but also acts as a neurotransmitter within the alerting system. Although first developed as a target for allergies, its known side effect of drowsiness has been used to help those with insomnia.

Diphenhydramine. Diphenhydramine is a first-generation antihistamine and acts as an inverse agonist at the H1 receptor, causing drowsiness and sleepiness. It is also a competitive antagonist of muscarinic acetylcholine receptor and, therefore, has anticholinergic effects. The half-life of diphenhydramine is 3.4 to 9.2 hours with an onset of action within 15 to 30 minutes. It is metabolized by CYP450 enzyme in the liver.

Diphenhydramine is available over the counter, making it a popular medication for patients to initially trial. Its effective dose starts at 25 mg and can be increased to 50 mg. Although there may be a very modest improvement in total sleep time,[35] it is outweighed by its multitude of adverse effects in the elderly.

Adverse effects. The long half-life of diphenhydramine causes grogginess, particularly at higher dosages. Because it also binds to muscarinic receptors, it can cause anticholinergic effects, such as dry mouth, difficulty urinating, confusion, memory impairment, and delirium. Currently, diphenhydramine is not recommended by American Geriatrics Society Beers Criteria or by the American Academy of Sleep Medicine to be given to elderly patients given higher risk of adverse effects.

Doxepin. Doxepin is a type of tricyclic antidepressant with sedative effects. Although its antidepressive effects are targeted via serotonin and norepinephrine receptors, at much lower doses doxepin can induce drowsiness and sleep via histaminergic neurons on selective H1 receptors. Its half-life is 6 to 8 hours and is metabolized by the liver via CYP2D6 and CYP2C19. Initial dosage starts at 3 mg and should not exceed 6 mg for the purposes of insomnia—higher doses are more beneficial for depression and anxiety. Overall, low-dose doxepin showed an increase in objective and subjective total sleep time as well as objective sleep efficiency.[26] In general, at such low doses doxepin is tolerable and lacks serious adverse effects, particularly on cognitive function and memory. Adverse effects of doxepin were similar to placebo, and no reported anticholinergic effects were observed at these lower dosages.[36]

Orexin and hypocretin antagonists

The orexin/hypocretin system, which was discovered in the late 1990s, is a major component of the brain's arousal systems. Orexin is a neuropeptide released by the lateral hypothalamus that regulates the sleep–wake cycle and sustains wakefulness. Antagonists to orexin receptors—orexin-1 and orexin-2—have become a pharmacologic target for inducing sleep and the treatment of insomnia. Two medications of this class are currently available on the US market. However, there are currently more dual orexin receptor antagonists being investigated.

Suvorexant (Belsomra)

The first orexin antagonist that was introduced into the market was suvorexant, marketed as Belsomra. It was approved by the FDA in 2014 for the treatment of both sleep-onset and sleep-maintenance insomnia. Its half-life is about 12 hours with an onset of action of 30 minutes. It is metabolized mostly in the liver by CYP3A4, so it should be prescribed with caution in patients on medications that can inhibit or induce the enzyme or those who have hepatic impairment. It acts as a potent and selective antagonist for both orexin receptors. Dosing starts at 5 mg before bedtime and should not exceed 20 mg. In general, suvorexant has shown good effects with increase in total sleep time, decrease in wake after sleep onset, and subjective sleep latency.[26]

Lemborexant (Dayvigo)

The newest orexin antagonist on the market is lemborexant (Dayvigo), which was approved by the FDA in 2019. Lemobrexant is more selective for orexin-2 receptors and dissociates rapidly compared with suvorexant.[37] The half-life of lemobrexant is 17 to 19 hours with a starting dose of 5 mg before bedtime, which can be increased to 10 mg/d, although this amount should be used with caution in the elderly. It is also metabolized by CYP3A4 and, like suvorexant, should be used with caution in medications that can inhibit or induce CYP3A4 as well as patients with liver disease. Similar to suvorexant, lemobrexant also improves total sleep time and sleep latency. In a randomized, double-blind trial, lemobrexant seemed to result in a significantly improved latency to sleep and sleep maintenance compared with both placebo and zolpidem.[38]

Adverse effects

In general, the most common adverse effects with dual orexin receptor antagonists were dizziness, nasopharyngitis, and headaches. There seems to be an increased risk for falls with suvorexant in a case control study,[39] but other studies have disputed this.[40]

Unlike other hypnotics, orexin antagonists do not seem to affect the respiratory system. A recent randomized, placebo-controlled study showed no difference in the apnea–hypopnea index and treatment-emergent events between those that used an orexin antagonist versus placebo.[41] This class of medication also seems to have no dependency or tolerance-inducing effects, unlike benzodiazepines and the Z drugs.[42]

Of note, dual orexin receptors are contraindicated in narcolepsy. Overall, orexin receptor antagonists are well tolerated and a safe drug to use in the elderly at the doses specified elsewhere in this article.

Melatonin and melatonin receptor agonists

Melatonin is a hormone produced by the pineal gland, which is released during the night. It is circadian driven and helps to induce sleep. Melatonin binds to two melatonin receptors. MT1 receptors help to both initiate and maintain sleep, and MT2 receptors help to regulate the circadian rhythm. Melatonin can be given directly or as an MT1 and MT2 receptor agonist.

Melatonin. Melatonin is a popular sleep aid. It is regarded as a dietary supplement, which makes it available over the counter, and it is not regulated by the FDA. There are many formulations of melatonin that often include various supplements such as vitamins or chamomile, and dosages can range from 0.3 mg to 60.0 mg. Because melatonin is not regulated by the FDA, the stated dosages on products may not reflect actual dosages, so stated dosages should be interpreted carefully. In Europe, there are several formulations that exist and have been regulated—immediate release tablets are available in doses of 0.3 to 0.5 mg and extended release is available in 2 mg.

Melatonin has shown a decrease in sleep-onset latency, but REM latency, total sleep time, and wake after sleep onset do not improve.[43] The half-life of melatonin is 1 hour, and the peak plasma concentration is achieved about 60 minutes after administration. Typically, particularly for elderly patients, doses should be started at the lowest dose. We recommended starting at 1 to 3 mg mg of melatonin for sleep. Higher dosages have clinical benefits in other sleep issues, such as circadian rhythm disorders and REM behavior disorders.

  Adverse effects Melatonin can often cause grogginess, irritability, nightmares, anxiety, and memory impairment, especially in much higher doses, but is otherwise well-tolerated at lower doses. Of note, there is very little potential for abuse, although high doses of melatonin should be avoided.

Ramelteon. Ramelteon is an MT1 and MT2 receptor agonist with a half-life of 1.0 to 2.5 hours and a rapid onset of action. It is metabolized by hepatic enzyme CYP1A2. Ramelteon has been shown to decrease subjective sleep onset latency and increase total sleep time.[26,44] The dosage of ramelteon for insomnia is 8 mg at bedtime. Although it has not been studied in elderly patients specifically, ramelteon has little effect on respiratory function and thus serves as a safe option for patients with chronic lung disease such as chronic obstructive pulmonary disease.[45]

  Adverse effects Ramelteon is generally well-tolerated and has little effects on balance, memory, and stability. When compared to zolpidem, ramelteon has a decreased risk for falls and injuries.[40] The most common side effects are dizziness, fatigue, and headache.

Other medications

Trazodone. Antidepressants have been used as a hypnotic medication. A recent metanalysis of several classes of antidepressants, including selective serotonin reuptake inhibitors, tricyclic antidepressants (eg, amitriptyline), and trazodone were compared. There is a lack of comprehensive clinical trials to investigate the efficacies of selective serotonin reuptake inhibitors and tricyclic antidepressants, including amitriptyline, which is commonly prescribed for insomnia.[46] However, trazodone did show short-term improvement in sleep quality as well as wake after sleep onset. It is a weak inhibitor of serotonin reuptake and an antagonist for several serotonin receptors. Lower trazodone doses at bedtime are indicated for insomnia, whereas higher doses of trazodone are more beneficial for depression. The half-life of trazodone is 7 to 10 hours, and it is metabolized by CYP3A4 so should be used with caution in patients with hepatic impairment and those taking concurrent CYP3A4 inducers or inhibitors. Trazodone should be started at 12.5 mg and be used in the lowest, effective dose. Dosages should not exceed 50 mg for the purposes of mitigating insomnia. Interestingly, an observational study in patients with secondary insomnia, including those with advanced cancer and depression, showed improvement in sleep and nightmares starting at 12.5 mg up to 50.0 mg.[47,48]

Adverse effects Trazodone has several adverse effects such as orthostatic hypotension and dizziness which increases the risk for falls in the elderly. It also may cause cognitive and memory impairment. More concerning, trazodone has the potential to prolong QT interval and induce ventricular tachycardia so should not be used with other QT prolonging medications or patients with underlying arrhythmias.

Cannabinoids

Marijuana has recently gained popularity particularly in the geriatric population, and is now legal in various states within the United States. It is composed of two active ingredients—tetrahydrocannabinol (THC) and cannabidiol (CBD). THC produces a psychoactive effect, causing the user to feel "high." CBD, in contrast, does not produce these effects, but has been advertised as a treatment for a variety of medical issues, such as anxiety and insomnia.

Cannabinoids in their various forms are often trialed by patients, who report anecdotal success in achieving sleep and in decreasing anxiety. However, CBD in the form of Epidiolex is the only FDA-approved formulation as a treatment for two rare forms of childhood epilepsy—Dravet syndrome and Lennox–Gastaut syndrome. Cannabinoids for the purposes of insomnia have not been fully regulated by the FDA. Cannabinoids can be consumed in a variety of different ways, including edibles, oils, smoking, and vaping. Of note, several case series have reported severe lung injury in the context of vaping THC oils,[49] and this practice should be discouraged.

There have been several trials that have investigated whether cannabinoids treat insomnia. Although a few small studies showed that THC helped to decrease sleep-onset latency, a recent systematic review and meta-analysis showed inconsistent

Table 3	
Common CYP3A4 inducers and inhibitors	
Inducers	**Inhibitors**
Antiepileptics: carbamazepine, fosphenytoin, phenytoin, phenobarbital	Azoles
	Amiodarone
	Diltiazem, verapamil
St. Johns wort	Protease inhibitors
Dexamethasone	Macrolide
Pioglitazone	H2 receptor antagonists (cimetidine)
	Selective serotonin reuptake inhibitors
	Grapefruit juice

results, citing that, across the studies, patients were heterogenous, and there was a high risk of bias.[50,51] At this time, there is an insufficient amount of evidence to conclude that cannabinoids treat insomnia.

SUMMARY

Insomnia remains a complex medical diagnosis and is difficult to treat. It affects about one-half of the geriatric population and has detrimental effects on health as well as economic costs to the health care system. A multifaceted and personalized approach to each patient is recommended and includes the treatment of potential underlying causes of insomnia such as comorbidities, medications, and cognitive behavioral therapy, as well as hypnotics. However, the challenge with treating insomnia in the geriatric population with hypnotics is balancing their intended effects with their potential adverse effects as well as drug interactions. Many hypnotics are metabolized by the liver enzyme, CYP3A4, and prescribers should be aware of potential inducers and inhibitors of the enzyme (**Table 3**).

Although nonbenzodiazepine Z drugs have been the mainstay of insomnia therapy for many years, like benzodiazepines they may cause devastating falls and injuries in the geriatric population. New pharmacologic targets have been developed that may have fewer adverse effects, including dual orexin receptor antagonists, and may be a better choice. As a general rule, hypnotics should always be started at the lowest dose and titrated up with caution, monitoring carefully for adverse effects.

CLINICS CARE POINTS

- Insomnia is often multifactorial, and the etiology includes secondary causes such as underlying psychiatric disease and sleep disordered breathing or adverse effects of medications.
- Hypnotics, particularly benzodiazepines and Z drugs like zolpidem, should be prescribed with caution in the elderly owing to adverse effects like falls, injuries, and parasomnias.
- Drug metabolism in the geriatric population is affected by age, drug interactions, and liver function, so hypnotics should always start with the lowest possible dose.
- As our understanding of sleep physiology grows, newer and more tolerable classes of hypnotics such as dual orexin receptor antagonists are available and should be considered.

DISCLOSURE

The authors have nothing to disclose.

REFERENCES

1. Shakespeare W, Shakespeare Memorial Company., Theater Playbills and Programs Collection (Library of Congress). Henry the Fourth, part 2. 1932.
2. Darien II. AAoS. The International Classification of Sleep Disorders—Third Edition (ICSD-3). American Academy of Sleep Medicine 2014.
3. Patel D, Steinberg J, Patel P. Insomnia in the elderly: a review. J Clin Sleep Med 2018;14(6):1017–24.
4. Tzuang M, Owusu JT, Huang J, et al. Associations of insomnia symptoms with subsequent health services use among community-Dwelling U.S. Older adults. Sleep 2020. https://doi.org/10.1093/sleep/zsaa251.

5. España RA, Scammell TE. Sleep neurobiology from a clinical perspective. Sleep 2011;34(7):845–58.
6. Olsen RW. Gaba. Neuropharmacology 2018;136(Pt A):10–22.
7. Liu J, Clough SJ, Hutchinson AJ, et al. MT1 and MT2 melatonin receptors: a therapeutic perspective. Annu Rev Pharmacol Toxicol 2016;56:361–83.
8. Vallières A, Morin CM, Guay B. Sequential combinations of drug and cognitive behavioral therapy for chronic insomnia: an exploratory study. Behav Res Ther 2005;43(12):1611–30.
9. Foral P, Knezevich J, Dewan N, et al. Medication-induced sleep disturbances. Consult Pharm 2011;26(6):414–25.
10. McCrae CS, Lichstein KL. Secondary insomnia: diagnostic challenges and intervention opportunities. Sleep Med Rev 2001;5(1):47–61.
11. López-Muñoz F, Ucha-Udabe R, Alamo C. The history of barbiturates a century after their clinical introduction. Neuropsychiatr Dis Treat 2005;1(4):329–43.
12. Kaufmann CN, Spira AP, Alexander GC, et al. Trends in prescribing of sedative-hypnotic medications in the USA: 1993-2010. Pharmacoepidemiol Drug Saf 2016;25(6):637–45.
13. Edinger JD, Arnedt JT, Bertisch SM, et al. Behavioral and psychological treatments for chronic insomnia disorder in adults: an American Academy of Sleep Medicine clinical practice guideline. J Clin Sleep Med 2020. https://doi.org/10.5664/jcsm.8986.
14. Sateia MJ, Buysse DJ, Krystal AD, et al. Clinical practice guideline for the pharmacologic treatment of chronic insomnia in adults: an American Academy of sleep medicine clinical practice guideline. J Clin Sleep Med 2017;13(2):307–49.
15. Bowie MW, Slattum PW. Pharmacodynamics in older adults: a review. Am J Geriatr Pharmacother 2007;5(3):263–303.
16. Panel BtAGSBCUE. American geriatrics society 2019 updated AGS Beers Criteria® for potentially inappropriate medication use in older adults. J Am Geriatr Soc 2019;67(4):674–94.
17. Vgontzas AN, Kales A, Bixler EO, et al. Temazepam 7.5 mg: effects on sleep in elderly insomniacs. Eur J Clin Pharmacol 1994;46(3):209–13.
18. Reeves RL. Comparison of triazolam, flurazepam, and placebo as hypnotics in geriatric patients with insomnia. J Clin Pharmacol 1977;17(5–6):319–23.
19. Carskadon MA, Seidel WF, Greenblatt DJ, et al. Daytime carryover of triazolam and flurazepam in elderly insomniacs. Sleep 1982;5(4):361–71.
20. Roehrs T, Zorick F, Wittig R, et al. Efficacy of a reduced triazolam dose in elderly insomniacs. Neurobiol Aging 1985;6(4):293–6.
21. Barker MJ, Greenwood KM, Jackson M, et al. Persistence of cognitive effects after withdrawal from long-term benzodiazepine use: a meta-analysis. Arch Clin Neuropsychol 2004;19(3):437–54.
22. Zhong G, Wang Y, Zhang Y, et al. Association between benzodiazepine use and dementia: a meta-analysis. PLoS One 2015;10(5):e0127836.
23. Higgitt A, Fonagy P, Lader M. The natural history of tolerance to the benzodiazepines. Psychol Med Monogr Suppl 1988;13:1–55.
24. Pétursson H. The benzodiazepine withdrawal syndrome. Addiction 1994;89(11):1455–9.
25. Lähteenmäki R, Neuvonen PJ, Puustinen J, et al. Withdrawal from long-term use of zopiclone, zolpidem and temazepam may improve perceived sleep and quality of life in older adults with primary insomnia. Basic Clin Pharmacol Toxicol 2019;124(3):330–40.

26. Chiu HY, Lee HC, Liu JW, et al. Comparative efficacy and safety of hypnotics for insomnia in older adults: a systematic review and network metaanalysis. Sleep 2020. https://doi.org/10.1093/sleep/zsaa260.

27. Montgomery P, Lilly J. Insomnia in the elderly. BMJ Clin Evid 2007;2007:1–16.

28. Treves N, Perlman A, Kolenberg Geron L, et al. Z-drugs and risk for falls and fractures in older adults-a systematic review and meta-analysis. Age Ageing 2018; 47(2):201–8.

29. Pressman MR. Sleep driving: sleepwalking variant or misuse of z-drugs? Sleep Med Rev 2011;15(5):285–92.

30. Harbourt K, Nevo ON, Zhang R, et al. Association of eszopiclone, zaleplon, or zolpidem with complex sleep behaviors resulting in serious injuries, including death. Pharmacoepidemiol Drug Saf 2020;29(6):684–91.

31. Victorri-Vigneau C, Laforgue EJ, Grall-Bronnec M, et al. Are seniors dependent on benzodiazepines? A National clinical survey of substance use disorder. Clin Pharmacol Ther 2020. https://doi.org/10.1002/cpt.2025.

32. Hajak G, Müller WE, Wittchen HU, et al. Abuse and dependence potential for the non-benzodiazepine hypnotics zolpidem and zopiclone: a review of case reports and epidemiological data. Addiction 2003;98(10):1371–8.

33. Choi JW, Lee J, Jung SJ, et al. Use of sedative-hypnotics and mortality: a population-Based retrospective cohort study. J Clin Sleep Med 2018;14(10): 1669–77.

34. Jaussent I, Ancelin ML, Berr C, et al. Hypnotics and mortality in an elderly general population: a 12-year prospective study. BMC Med 2013;11:212.

35. Morin CM, Koetter U, Bastien C, et al. Valerian-hops combination and diphenhydramine for treating insomnia: a randomized placebo-controlled clinical trial. Sleep 2005;28(11):1465–71.

36. Katwala J, Kumar A, Seipal J, et al. Therapeutic rationale for low dose doxepin in insomnia patients. Asian Pac J Trop Dis 2013;3(4):331–6.

37. Murphy P, Moline M, Mayleben D, et al. Lemborexant, A dual orexin receptor antagonist (DORA) for the treatment of insomnia disorder: results from a Bayesian, Adaptive, randomized, double-blind, placebo-controlled study. J Clin Sleep Med 2017;13(11):1289–99.

38. Rosenberg R, Murphy P, Zammit G, et al. Comparison of lemborexant with placebo and zolpidem Tartrate extended release for the treatment of older adults with insomnia disorder: a phase 3 randomized clinical trial. JAMA Netw Open 2019;2(12):e1918254.

39. Ishibashi Y, Nishitani R, Shimura A, et al. Non-GABA sleep medications, suvorexant as risk factors for falls: case-control and case-crossover study. PLoS One 2020;15(9):e0238723.

40. Torii H, Ando M, Tomita H, et al. Association of hypnotic drug use with fall Incidents in hospitalized elderly patients: a case-crossover study. Biol Pharm Bull 2020;43(6):925–31.

41. Cheng JY, Filippov G, Moline M, et al. Respiratory safety of lemborexant in healthy adult and elderly subjects with mild obstructive sleep apnea: a randomized, double-blind, placebo-controlled, crossover study. J Sleep Res 2020;29(4): e13021.

42. Muehlan C, Vaillant C, Zenklusen I, et al. Clinical pharmacology, efficacy, and safety of orexin receptor antagonists for the treatment of insomnia disorders. Expert Opin Drug Metab Toxicol 2020;16(11):1063–78.

43. Brzezinski A, Vangel MG, Wurtman RJ, et al. Effects of exogenous melatonin on sleep: a meta-analysis. Sleep Med Rev 2005;9(1):41–50.

44. Roth T, Seiden D, Sainati S, et al. Effects of ramelteon on patient-reported sleep latency in older adults with chronic insomnia. Sleep Med 2006;7(4):312–8.
45. Roth T. Hypnotic use for insomnia management in chronic obstructive pulmonary disease. Sleep Med 2009;10(1):19–25.
46. Everitt H, Baldwin DS, Stuart B, et al. Antidepressants for insomnia in adults. Cochrane Database Syst Rev 2018;5:CD010753.
47. Tanimukai H, Murai T, Okazaki N, et al. An observational study of insomnia and nightmare treated with trazodone in patients with advanced cancer. Am J Hosp Palliat Care 2013;30(4):359–62.
48. Saletu-Zyhlarz GM, Anderer P, Arnold O, et al. Confirmation of the neurophysiologically predicted therapeutic effects of trazodone on its target symptoms depression, anxiety and insomnia by postmarketing clinical studies with a controlled-release formulation in depressed outpatients. Neuropsychobiology 2003;48(4):194–208.
49. Fryman C, Lou B, Weber AG, et al. Acute respiratory failure associated with vaping. Chest 2020;157(3):e63–8.
50. Bhagavan C, Kung S, Doppen M, et al. Cannabinoids in the treatment of insomnia disorder: a systematic review and meta-analysis. CNS Drugs 2020;34(12): 1217–28.
51. Suraev AS, Marshall NS, Vandrey R, et al. Cannabinoid therapies in the management of sleep disorders: a systematic review of preclinical and clinical studies. Sleep Med Rev 2020;53:101339.

Obstructive Sleep Apnea

Treatment with Positive Airway Pressure

Steven H. Feinsilver, MD

KEYWORDS

- CPAP • BilevelPAP • APAP • Obstructive sleep apnea • Sleepiness
- Cardiovascular outcomes • Quality of life • Hypertension

KEY POINTS

- PAP remains the most effective treatment for sleep apnea.
- Recent advances including autotitrating machines have made this treatment easier for both clinician and patient.
- Interface selection is key to patient comfort and compliance.
- Benefits of treatment include amelioration of sleepiness and cardiovascular risk.

The original description of the use of positive airway pressure (PAP) as a "pneumatic splint" for the upper airway to treat sleep-disordered breathing is now 40 years old.[1] This has become the most reliably effective and fastest form of therapy for this condition, except perhaps for tracheotomy, which is very rarely indicated. With continuing technological advances, this treatment has evolved to be easier and easier both for the practitioner to prescribe and for the patient to use. With attention to detail, most patients with significant sleep-disordered breathing can be made comfortable with this treatment. In elderly individuals there may be some specific challenges, but this remains the mainstay of therapy as in other adults. This article reviews the basics of PAP treatment and where its use and indications may vary between elderly individuals and other adults.

POSITIVE AIRWAY PRESSURE: CONTINUOUS POSITIVE AIRWAY PRESSURE, BILEVEL POSITIVE AIRWAY PRESSURE, AUTO-TITRATING POSITIVE AIRWAY PRESSURE

PAP may include continuous positive airway pressure (CPAP), bilevel PAP, auto-titrating PAP (APAP), and assisted servo-ventilation (ASV) (**Table 1**). Conventional CPAP consists of a compressor with pressure feedback that delivers as much flow as is necessary to maintain a constant positive pressure throughout the respiratory cycle. CPAP has become smaller, completely quiet, and smarter over the years. It is now routine for most machines to monitor and record hours of use (adherence/compliance) and apnea hypopnea index (AHI) (efficacy) while the machine is in use, in addition to

Zucker School of Medicine at Hofstra Northwell Health, Lenox Hill Hospital, New York, NY, USA
E-mail address: sfeinsil@northwell.edu

Clin Geriatr Med 37 (2021) 417–427
https://doi.org/10.1016/j.cger.2021.04.004
0749-0690/21/© 2021 Elsevier Inc. All rights reserved.

Table 1
Modes of positive airway pressure (PAP)

Abbreviation	Mode	Mechanism of Action
CPAP	Constant positive airway pressure	Set pressure
Bilevel PAP	Bilevel positive airway pressure	Independently set inspiratory and expiratory pressures
APAP	Automatic positive airway pressure	Set range of pressures: machine adjusts based on patient's breathing
ASV	Assisted servo-ventilation	Machine adjusts pressure based on minute ventilation: rarely used for obstructive sleep apnea
EPR or C-flex	Expiratory pressure relief (added feature, not a stand-alone mode)	Pressure reduced in early part of expiration; option on PAP machines, may improve patient comfort

data about interface leak. These data are uploaded via the Internet for the clinician to use to guide treatment. This has revolutionized treatment monitoring and should now be considered standard of care.

Bilevel PAP is a modification of CPAP originally designed to improve patient comfort by using separate pressures for inspiration and expiration. The expectation was that lower pressures on expiration would be more comfortable; however, 2 randomized trials showed no difference in compliance.[2,3] There are some patients who are not compliant with CPAP who may do better with bilevel PAP,[4,5] and in one study improved adherence was seen in patients who were older, had more severe apnea, concomitant heart failure, or chronic obstructive pulmonary disease.[6] Bilevel PAP can also be used as a form of noninvasive ventilation.

APAP uses proprietary algorithms to measure and respond to obstructive apnea events by adjusting pressure up or down throughout the night as needed. This, in theory at least, allows for optimally effective pressure, as the pressure requirement varies with sleep position, stage of sleep, and perhaps other variables during the night. For some patients who find it difficult to tolerate the fixed CPAP pressure needed for treating apnea in all positions and sleep stages, this allows lower pressures for at least some of the night. The use of APAP might also be an advantage for patients whose weight, rhinitis due to seasonal allergies, and alcohol use might be expected to vary from night to night. Originally intended for initiation of PAP, this is now frequently used for long-term treatment. This is thought not to be advisable in patients with significant cardiac or respiratory illness. Most studies have found that efficacy of APAP and CPAP were equivalent, with some showing a small advantage for adherence, quality of life, or sleepiness for APAP over CPAP.[7,8] Originally significantly more expensive, the difference in cost between CPAP and APAP is now minimal, and APAP has become routine in many practices.

The American Academy of Sleep Medicine (AASM) 2019 guidelines recommend either initiation of PAP with APAP at home or CPAP titration in a sleep center, and long-term use of either CPAP or APAP.[9] Bilevel PAP is not recommended for the routine treatment of obstructive sleep apnea (OSA). ASV adjusts PAP to a target level of ventilation, mostly to treat central sleep apnea, which is not discussed further here.

INDICATIONS FOR POSITIVE AIRWAY PRESSURE

PAP treatment is the treatment of choice for patients with moderate to severe OSA; however, it is not always obvious who needs this treatment along the spectrum of sleep-disordered breathing from simple snoring to severe OSA. CPAP can be successful in eliminating snoring, but few would find this worthwhile, and there is no evidence that simple snoring is a disease or has significant morbidity. In the United States, the Centers for Medicare and Medicaid Services (CMS) permits treatment of moderate to severe sleep apnea as defined by an AHI of at least 15, or at least 5 in patients with "excessive daytime sleepiness, impaired cognition, mood disorders or insomnia, or documented hypertension, ischemic heart disease, or history of stroke."[10] Note that CMS requires a 4% oxygen desaturation to define a hypopnea. CMS also will not reimburse for PAP treatment unless the patient is shown to use the device at least 70% of nights for at least 4 hours per night.

For patients with mild sleep apnea, treatment may not always be required. There is no general consensus regarding the benefit of treatment, or even on the definition of mild apnea. However, in a recent randomized controlled trial (the MERGE study), 3 months of CPAP did appear to improve quality of life.[11]

INITIATING TREATMENT

Until recently, standard practice was to determine the best PAP pressure by titration in a sleep center during polysomnography. Guidelines from a task force of the AASM were published in 2008.[12] After patient education and fitting of a comfortable mask interface, pressure is begun at 4 cm water pressure and increased at 5 minutes or longer intervals for 2 apneas, 3 hypopneas, at least 3 minutes of snoring, or 5 or more respiratory effort related arousals. An important paper by Montserrat and colleagues[13] showed that with increasing PAP pressure, snoring, apneas and hypopneas, and then arousals are eliminated. Higher pressures are needed to treat inspiratory flow limitation as measured by the shape of the inspiratory flow curve. The elimination of flow limitation as seen on the airflow signal from the CPAP mask is thought to imply optimal titration. This is also the signal used for most auto-titrating machines.

"Split-night" studies, which combine diagnosis and treatment on the same night in the sleep laboratory, may be useful for lowering cost and expediting treatment. Treatment with CPAP is begun if the AHI is at least 40 events per hour during the first 2 hours of the study and at least 3 hours remain for CPAP titration. In general, studies show equivalence of split-night and full-night studies in determining the best CPAP pressure, although some studies will be incompletely successful and worse sleep quality of split-night studies could impact CPAP acceptance and compliance.[14,15]

INTERFACE SELECTION

The interface ("mask") used to deliver pressure is not a trivial decision. Probably the most important issue in patient acceptance of PAP therapy is the interface. These come in 3 basic types: a more or less triangular nasal mask that covers only the nose, a full face (oronasal) mask that covers both nose and mouth, and an under the nose device with a cushion that presses against the nostrils to make a seal. The engineering of interfaces has dramatically improved over the years, and they are now available in a wide variety of sizes and shapes. Fit and comfort of the interface is critical, and patients often need to try several before optimal comfort is achieved. All interfaces are designed to leak, as they vent expired air. CPAP devices are designed to increase flow to compensate for leakage to a large extent, and this information will be available when the CPAP machine is downloaded after use. High leakage may exceed the capacity of the device to compensate and be effective, and large leaks may cause excessive noise and dryness. Leakage of air around the eyes is particularly troublesome. In general, nasal interfaces are to be preferred over full face masks, which may be less comfortable and require higher pressures.[16] Full face masks should be reserved for those with chronic nasal congestion.

EXPIRATORY PRESSURE REDUCTION

Positive pressure on inspiration is inherently more comfortable than expiring against positive pressure. A common option on CPAP machines reduces pressure in the beginning of expiration to attempt to make PAP more comfortable (marketed as C-Flex or A-Flex or EPR). In one study, there were no significant differences in improvements in sleepiness or quality of life compared with standard CPAP,[17] although it was judged more comfortable in another trial.[18] This could be used if felt to be subjectively better by the patient.

ADHERENCE TO CONTINUOUS POSITIVE AIRWAY PRESSURE THERAPY

For several years, most insurance companies, beginning with Medicare, have required a minimum usage of CPAP to approve reimbursement, generally at least 4 hours per night for 70% of nights for 30 days in the first 90 days after starting treatment. In addition to this financial requirement, early experience with CPAP has been shown to influence long-term adherence to treatment.[19] Acceptance of therapy requires attention to patient education and proper mask fit and comfort. Initial nasal irritation is common, usually responding to treatment with proper humidification and often the use of topical nasal corticosteroids. Both efficacy and usage data are now routinely available to the clinician and need to be followed closely in the initial few months of treatment.

There have been several trials to see if hypnotic use during therapy initiation might be of benefit. Eszopiclone for CPAP titration helped in one study,[20] zolpidem for 2 weeks did not help,[21] eszopiclone for 2 weeks of initial use helped in another study.[22] In none of these studies did treatment appear to be harmful, suggesting this might at least occasionally be useful, perhaps especially in elderly subjects who are more prone to fragmented sleep, with the caveat that lower doses should be used.

Acceptance and compliance with long-term treatment with CPAP are critical but problematic. It is possible that improvements in comfort and monitoring are improving CPAP usage, but in a 1999 study, 30% of patients refused this treatment at onset, and another 25% discontinued in 1 year.[23] Lower socioeconomic status, depression, anxiety, history of stroke, and sinusitis predict worse adherence. Physiologic factors including AHI, body mass index, and sleepiness only weakly predict adherence; the subjective perception of benefit by the patient may be more important.[24,25] Older age does not itself appear to be predictive of success or failure.[26]

BENEFITS OF CONTINUOUS POSITIVE AIRWAY PRESSURE THERAPY
Daytime Sleepiness and Cognitive Function

With successful use of CPAP, sleep quality and sleepiness improve within days, reaching a plateau in approximately 2 weeks. One important measure of this is driving performance, which can improve within several days of treatment when assessed on driving simulators.[27,28] The minimal amount of CPAP use required to improve daytime sleepiness is uncertain and likely varies among patients. A 2007 study by Weaver and colleagues[29] looked at the relationship between hours of CPAP use and daytime functioning. Thresholds above which further improvements were less likely relative to nightly duration of CPAP use were identified for various outcome measures. For the Epworth Sleepiness Scale score this was 4 hours, Multiple Sleep Latency Test 6 hours, and Functional Outcomes associated with Sleepiness Questionnaire (FOSQ) 7.5 hours. FOSQ is a sleep-specific questionnaire assessing the impact of sleep disturbance on daily life. A linear dose–response relationship between increased use and normalcy was shown for objective and subjective daytime sleepiness, reaching a maximum at 7 hours of use for functional status.

As most patients have symptoms for years before seeking treatment, it is certainly reasonable to assume that there might be permanent consequences of sleep apnea that are not completely reversible. The lack of complete resolution of neurocognitive defects may be related to effects of intermittent hypoxia as seen in animal studies.[30] In a study of 17 patients with severe apnea (AHI >30) and 15 matched controls, MRI neuroimaging of patients with apnea showed focal reductions in gray matter volume, which improved with 3 months of CPAP treatment, with parallel improvements in memory, attention, and executive functioning.[31] Clearly, however, some patients remain significantly sleepy and may have cognitive deficits despite optimal treatment. Antic and colleagues,[32] in 141 patients with moderate to severe apnea, showed substantial and dose-related (hours of CPAP use) improvement in sleepiness (Epworth score) and FOSQ. However, even at optimal CPAP adherence (>7 hours of use per night), nearly 20% did not normalize Epworth scores, 32% did not have normal maintenance of wakefulness test, and more than 50% had an abnormal FOSQ. The Apnea Positive Pressure Long-term Efficacy Study (APPLES) was designed to investigate the long-term neurocognitive benefits of CPAP treatment.[33] This was a multicenter 6-month randomized trial involving more than 1000 patients with sham-CPAP controls. Measurements of sleepiness improved, but the only neurocognitive tests to improve involved executive and frontal function where the effect appeared transient. Tests of learning and memory, and tests for attention and psychomotor function did not significantly change. In a randomized controlled trial in 278 elderly subjects (>65 years of age) CPAP use did significantly improve sleepiness compared with best supportive care.[34]

The prevalence of residual sleepiness in patients well treated with CPAP has been estimated as high as 12%.[35] For these patients, pharmacologic treatment may be helpful. The wakefulness promoting agent modafinil has been studied and has been approved for this indication.[36] More recently, the selective dopamine and norepinephrine reuptake inhibitor solriamfetol has also been found to be effective and has been approved.[37] However, it must be stressed that optimal CPAP compliance as well as sleep hygiene need to be established first as much as possible before any chronic medication is considered.

Cognitive function is of particular importance to the elderly population. In a recent meta-analysis of 4 trials with a total of 680 patients 65 years of age or older, Labarca and colleagues[38] showed overall improvements in sleepiness and health-related quality of life, with a slight improvement in neurocognitive function, but rated the quality of evidence as low to very low. At least as important is the possibility that treating sleep-disordered breathing could reduce the progression of cognitive decline. In a study by Osorio and colleagues,[39] the presence of sleep-disordered breathing was associated with an earlier age of onset of minimal cognitive impairment (MCI) or dementia, and CPAP use was possibly associated with delayed progression. In a nonrandomized study, CPAP adherence appeared to slow cognitive impairment over 1 year in patients with MCI.[40]

Mood and Affect

Depression is common in sleep disorders generally, and up to 25% of patients with sleep apnea described themselves as depressed.[41] There is evidence that CPAP benefits patients with mood disturbances.[42,43] In a study specifically of those older than 70 years, symptoms of both depression and anxiety were significantly improved after 3 months of CPAP versus no CPAP.[44] Two randomized, open label studies have looked at the effect of CPAP treatment in elderly individuals. Martinez-Garcia and colleagues[45] reported improvement in quality of life, anxiety, depression, and some neurocognitive testing with CPAP treatment for 3 months. A study by Ponce and colleagues[46] showed improvement in Epworth Sleepiness Scores and measures of quality of life, with no effect on blood pressure or neurocognitive tests.

Cardiovascular Disease, Hypertension, and Stroke

OSA is a complex phenomenon involving 3 physiologic events: intermittent hypoxia and reoxygenation, sleep disruption, and negative intrathoracic pressures. All of these may contribute to cardiovascular dysfunction and risk. Hypertension, coronary disease, arrhythmias, heart failure, and stroke have all been linked to OSA. Epidemiology is difficult to interpret, as the risk factors for sleep apnea (age, male gender, obesity) overlap with cardiovascular risk factors. However, data from the Sleep Heart Health Study of healthy subjects older than 40 years showed a higher prevalence of stroke, heart failure, and coronary disease with even small increases in AHI when corrected for other risks.[47]

In patients with OSA, CPAP use has a modest but significant effect on hypertension: 2 to 3 mm Hg in one study.[48] However, it is considered possibly the most common cause of resistant hypertension (defined as uncontrolled with 3 medications).[49] Significant improvement in blood pressure control in patients with resistant hypertension was seen with CPAP treatment in 2 studies.[50,51]

Evidence for CPAP treatment preventing cardiovascular disease is less certain. Treatment has been associated with reduced subclinical heart disease,[52,53] and in a 10-year, nonrandomized, observational study reduced the number of cerebrovascular and coronary events in 1347 men.[54] In the SAVE trial, however, patients with preexisting cardiovascular disease without significant sleepiness were randomized to CPAP or best care for a mean of 3.7 years and failed to show an effect of CPAP on further cardiovascular events.[55]

It is now well recognized that treatment of sleep apnea reduces the recurrence of atrial fibrillation after cardioversion or ablation,[56,57] and patients with this arrhythmia should be screened for possible sleep apnea.

Table 2
Benefits of continuous positive airway pressure treatment

Benefit	In Adults	In Elderly
Reduced sleepiness	Proven	Proven
Improved mood, affect	Proven	Proven
Blood pressure control	Proven	Probable
Cardiovascular risk	Likely	Likely
Atrial fibrillation control	Proven	Proven
Mortality	Probable	Probable

Sleep apnea is a common risk factor for stroke and transient ischemic attacks.[58] There is increasing evidence that treatment of sleep apnea with CPAP may improve patient outcomes after stroke.[59,60]

Mortality

The most compelling reason to treat OSA with CPAP would be reduced mortality. In an observational study of more than 2000 patients with a mean age of 56, CPAP use was associated with a lower risk of cardiovascular events and death.[61] In a study restricted to patients 65 or older, increased mortality was seen for those untreated with severe OSA (hazard ratio [HR] 2.25, confidence interval [CI] 1.41–3.61), as well as those with mild to moderate OSA (HR 1.38, CI 0.73–2.64).[62] Even in very elderly individuals (80 or older), CPAP treatment for those with AHI 20 or higher reduced mortality.[63]

SUMMARY

CPAP remains the most successful treatment for sleep-disordered breathing despite challenges with patient comfort and compliance. Recent technological advances have made treatment simpler, often with the use of automated pressure generators, more comfortable with a widening selection of interfaces, and easier to manage with CPAP use and efficacy data recorded night by night and available over the Internet. Although data about treatment outcomes are still emerging, there is every reason to believe that CPAP treatment represents significant clinical benefit to those with moderate to severe OSA, including elderly individuals. A summary of an estimate of outcomes data is shown in **Table 2**.

CLINICS CARE POINTS

- In the elderly as in other patients, CPAP remains the most reliably effective treatment for sleep apnea.
- Treatment leads to improved quality of life.
- It is likely, if not proven, that treatment leads to benefits in cardiovascular risk and mortality.

REFERENCES

1. Sullivan C, Issa F, Berthon-Jones M, et al. Reversal of obstructive sleep apnea by continuous positive airway pressure applied through the nares. Lancet 1981;1:862–5.
2. Gay PC, Herold DL, Olson EJ. A randomized, double blind clinical trial comparing continuous positive airway pressure with a novel bilevel pressure system for treatment of obstructive sleep apnea syndrome. Sleep 2003;26:864–9.
3. Blau A, Minx M, Decker B, et al. Respiration and sleep in OSA patients treated with CPAP vs. auto bilevel pressure relief-pap. Sleep 2008;31:A191.
4. Schafer H, Ewig S, Hasper E, et al. Failure of CPAP therapy in obstructive sleep apnoea syndrome: predictive factors and treatment with bilevel-positive airway pressure. Respir Med 1998;92:208–15.
5. Ballard RD, Gay PC, Strollo PJ. Interventions to improve compliance in sleep apnea patients previously non-compliant with continuous positive airway pressure. J Clin Sleep Med 2007;3:706–12.
6. Schwartz SW, Rosas J, Iannacone MR, et al. Correlates of a prescription for bilevel positive airway pressure for treatment of obstructive sleep apnea among veterans. J Clin Sleep Med 2013;9(4):327–35.

7. Ayas NT, Patel SR, Malhotra A, et al. Auto-titrating versus standard continuous positive airway pressure for the treatment of obstructive sleep apnea. Sleep 2004;27:249.

8. Bloch KE, Huber F, Furian M, et al. Autoadjusted versus fixed CPAP for obstructive sleep apnoea: a multicenter, randomized equivalence trial. Thorax 2018; 73:174.

9. Patil SP, Ayappa IA, Caples SM, et al. Treatment of adult obstructive sleep apnea with positive airway pressure: an AASM clinical practice guideline. J Clin Sleep Med 2019;15(2):335–43.

10. Center for Medicare and Medicaid Services. Pub 100-03, Medicare National Coverage Determinations. Available at: https://www.cms.gov/Regulations-and-Guidance/Guidance/Manuals/Internet-Only-Manuals-IOMs-Items/CMS014961.

11. Wimms AJ, Turnbull CD, McMillan A, et al. Continuous positive airway pressure versus standard of care for the treatment of people with mild obstructive sleep apnoea (MERGE): a multicenter, randomized controlled trial. Lancet Resp Med 2020;8:349–58.

12. Kushida CA, Kushida CA, Berry RB, et al. Positive airway pressure initiation: a randomized controlled trial to assess the impact of therapy mode and titration process on efficacy, adherence, and outcomes. Sleep 2010;34(8):1083–92.

13. Montserrat JM, Ballester E, Olivi H, et al. Timecourse of stepwise CPAP titration. Behavior of respiratory and neurologic variables. Am J Respir Crit Care Med 1995;152:1854–9.

14. McArdle N, Grove A, Devereux G, et al. Split night versus full night studies for sleep apnoea/hypopnea syndrome. Eur Respir J 2000;15:670–5.

15. Sanders MH, Costantino JP, Strollo PJ, et al. The impact of one night polysomnography for diagnosis and positive pressure therapy titration on treatment acceptance and appearance in sleep apnea/hypopnea. Sleep 2000;23:17–24.

16. Genta PR, Kaminska M, Edwards BA, et al. The importance of mask selection on CPAP outcomes for obstructive sleep apnea. Ann ATS 2020;17:1177–85.

17. Bakker J, Campbell A, Neill A. Randomized controlled trial comparing flexible and continuous positive pressure airway pressure delivery: effects on compliance, objective and subjective sleepiness and vigilance. Sleep 2010;33(4): 523–9.

18. Wenzel M, Kerl J, Dellweg D. Expiratory pressure reduction (C-Flex method) versus fixed CPAP in the therapy for obstructive sleep apnea. Pneumonologie 2007;61:692–5.

19. Lewis K, SealeL L, Bartle IE, et al. Early predictors of CPAP use for the treatment of obstructive sleep apnea. Sleep 2004;27:134–8.

20. Lettieri CJ, Collen JF, Eliasson AH, et al. Sedative use during CPAP titration improves subsequent compliance. Chest 2009;136:1263–8.

21. Bradshaw DA, Ruff GA, Murphy DP. An oral hypnotic does not improve CPAP compliance in men with obstructive sleep apnea. Chest 2006;130:1369.

22. Lettieri CA, Sah AA, Holley AB, et al. Effects of a short course of eszopiclone on CPAP adherence: a randomized trial. Ann Int Med 2009;151:696–702.

23. McArdle N, Devereux G, Heidarnejad H, et al. Long-term use of CPAP therapy for sleep apnea/hypopnea syndrome. Am J Respir Crit Care Med 1999;159(4 Pt 1): 1108–14.

24. Olsen S, Smith S, Oei T, et al. Health belief model predicts adherence to CPAP before experience with CPAP. Eur Respir J 2008;32:710–7.

25. Drake CL, Day R, Hudgel D, et al. Sleep during titration predicts CPAP compliance. Sleep 2003;26:308–11.

26. Weaver TE, Chassens ER. CPAP treatment of sleep apnea in older adults. Sleep Med Rev 2007;11:99–111.

27. George CF. Reduction in motor vehicle collisions following treatment of sleep apnoea with nasal CPAP. Thorax 2001;56:508–12.

28. Turkington PM, Sircar M, Saralaya D, et al. Time course of changes in driving simulator performance with and without treatment in patients with sleep apnoea hypopnea syndrome. Thorax 2004;59:56–9.

29. Weaver TE, Maislin G, Dinges DF, et al. Relationship between hours of CPAP use and achieving normal levels of sleepiness and daily functioning. Sleep 2007; 30(6):711–9.

30. Veasey S, Davis C, Fenik P, et al. Long-term intermittent hypoxia in mice: protracted hypersomnolence with oxidative injury to sleep-wake brain regions. Sleep 2004;27:194–201.

31. Canessa N, Castronovo V, Cappa SF, et al. Obstructive sleep apnea: brain structural changes and neurocognitive function before and after treatment. Am J Respir Crit Care Med 2011;183:1419–26.

32. Antic NA, Catcheside P, Buchan C, et al. The effect of CPAP in normalizing daytime sleepiness, quality of life, and neurocognitive function in patients with moderate to severe OSA. Sleep 2011;34(1):111–9.

33. Kushida CA, Nichols DA, Holmes TH, et al. Effects of continuous positive airway pressure on neurocognitive function in obstructive sleep apnea patients: the Apnea Positive Pressure Long-term Efficacy Study (APPLES). Sleep 2012;35(12): 1593–602.

34. McMillan A, Bratton DJ, Faria R, et al. A multicenter randomised controlled trial and economic evaluation of CPAP for the treatment of obstructive sleep apnoea syndrome in older people: predict. Health Technol Assess 2015;19:40.

35. Pépin J-L, Viot-Blanc V, Escourrou P, et al. Prevalence of residual excessive sleepiness in CPAP-treated sleep apnoea patients: the French multicentre study. Eur Respir J 2009;33:1062–7.

36. Black J, Hirshkowitz M. Modafinil for the treatment of residual excessive sleepiness in nasal CPAP treated obstructive sleep apnea/hypopnea syndrome. Sleep 2005;28:464–71.

37. Schweitzer PK, Rosenberg R, Zammit GK, et al, TONES 3 Study Investigators. Solriamfetol for excessive sleepiness in obstructive sleep apnea (TONES 3). A randomized controlled trial. Am J Respir Crit Care Med 2019;199(11):1421–31.

38. Labarca G, Saavedra D, Dreyse J, et al. Efficacy of CPAP for improvements in sleepiness, cognition, mood, and quality of life in elderly patients with OSA. Chest 2020;158(2):751–64.

39. Osorio RS, Gumb T, Pirraglia E, et al. Sleep-disordered breathing advances cognitive decline in the elderly. Neurology 2015;84:1964–71.

40. Richards KC, Gooneratne N, Dicicco B, et al. CPAP adherence may slow 1-year cognitive decline in older adults with mild cognitive impairment and apnea. J Am Geriatr Soc 2019;67(3):558–64.

41. Mendelson W. Depression in sleep apnea patients. Sleep Res 1992;21:230.

42. Gagnadoux F, Le Vaillant M, Goupil F, et al. Depressive symptoms before and after long-term CPAP therapy in patients with sleep apnea. Chest 2014;145: 1025–31.

43. Edwards C, Mukherjee S, Simpson L, et al. Depressive symptoms before and after treatment of obstructive sleep apnea in men and women. J Clin Sleep Med 2015;11:1029–38.

44. Kerner NA, Roose SP. Obstructive sleep apnea is linked to depression and cognitive impairment: evidence and potential mechanisms. Am J Geriatr Psychiatry 2016;24(6):496–508.
45. Martínez-García MÁ, Chiner E, Hernández L, et al. Spanish Sleep Network. Obstructive sleep apnoea in the elderly: role of continuous positive airway pressure treatment. Eur Respir J 2015;46(1):142–51.
46. Ponce S, Pastor E, Orosa B, et al, on behalf the Sleep Respiratory Disorders Group of the Sociedad Valenciana de Neumología. The role of CPAP treatment in elderly patients with moderate obstructive sleep apnoea: a multicentre randomised controlled trial. Eur Respir J 2019;54(2):1900518.
47. Shahar E, Whitney CW, Redline S, et al. Sleep disordered breathing and cardiovascular disease. Am J Respir Crit Care Med 2001;163:19–25.
48. Alajmi M, Mulgrew AT, Fox J, et al. Impact of CPAP therapy on blood pressure in patients with obstructive sleep apnea hypopnea: a meta-analysis of randomized clinical trials. Lung 2007;185(2):67–72.
49. Pedrosa RP, Drager LF, Gonzaga CC, et al. Obstructive sleep apnea: the most common secondary cause of hypertension associated with resistant hypertension. Hypertension 2011;58(5):811–7.
50. Martinez-Garcia M-A, Capote F, Campos-Rodriguez F, et al. Effect of CPAP on blood pressure in patients with obstructive sleep apnea and resistant hypertension, the HIPARCO trial. JAMA 2013;310(22):2407–15.
51. Pedrosa RP, Drager LF, dePaula LKG, et al. Effects o OSA treatment on BP in patients with resistant hypertension, a randomized trial. Chest 2013;144(5):1487–94.
52. Drager LF, Bortolotto LA, Figueiredo AC, et al. Effects of CPAP on early signs of atherosclerosis in OSA. Am J Respir Crit Care Med 2007;176:706–12.
53. Sharma SK, Agarwal S, Damodaran D, et al. CPAP for the metabolic syndrome in patients with obstructive sleep apnea. N Engl J Med 2011;365(24):2277–86.
54. Marin JM, Carrizo SJ, Vicente E, et al. Long-term cardiovascular outcomes in men with or without treatment with CPAP: an observational study. Lancet 2005;365(9464):1046–53.
55. McEvoy RD, Antic NA, Heeley E, et al. SAVE Investigators and Coordinators. CPAP for prevention of cardiovascular events in obstructive sleep apnea. N Engl J Med 2016;375(10):919–31.
56. Kanagala R, Murali NS, Friedman PA, et al. Obstructive sleep apnea and the recurrence of atrial fibrillation. Circulation 2003;107:2589–94.
57. Fein AS, Shvilkin A, Shah D, et al. Treatment of obstructive sleep apnea reduces the risk of atrial fibrillation recurrence after catheter ablation. J Am Coll Cardiol 2013;62(4):300–5.
58. Yaggi HK, Concato J, Kernan WN, et al. Obstructive sleep apnea as a risk factor for stroke and death. N Engl J Med 2005;353(19):2034–41.
59. Ren L, Wang K, Shen H, et al. Effects of continuous positive airway pressure (CPAP) therapy on neurological and functional rehabilitation in Basal Ganglia Stroke patients with obstructive sleep apnea: a prospective multicenter study. Medicine (Baltimore) 2019;98(28):e16344.
60. Ryan CM, Bayley M, Green R, et al. Influence of CPAP on outcomes of rehabilitation in stroke patients with OSA. Stroke 2011;42(4):1062–7.
61. Myllylä M, Hammais A, Stepanov M, et al. Nonfatal and fatal cardiovascular disease events in CPAP compliant obstructive sleep apnea patients. Sleep Breath 2019;23(4):1209–17.

62. Martínez-García MA, Campos-Rodríguez F, Catalán-Serra P, et al. Cardiovascular mortality in obstructive sleep apnea in the elderly: role of long-term continuous positive airway pressure treatment: a prospective observational study. Am J Respir Crit Care Med 2012;186(9):909–16.
63. Lopez-Padilla D, Alonso-Moralejo R, Martinez-Garcia MA, et al. Continuous positive airway pressure and survival of very elderly persons with moderate to severe obstructive sleep apnea Sleep. Medicine 2016;19:23–9.

Obstructive Sleep Apnea
Non–positive Airway Pressure Treatments

Maria V. Suurna, MD[a], Ana C. Krieger, MD, MPH[b],*

KEYWORDS

- Obstructive sleep apnea • Sleep apnea surgery • Oral appliance
- Hypoglossal nerve stimulation • Central apnea • Phrenic nerve stimulation

KEY POINTS

- Untreated obstructive sleep apnea (OSA) can lead to significant morbidity and mortality.
- Alternatives to positive airway pressure (PAP) treatment are effective in treatment of OSA.
- Hypoglossal nerve stimulation is an alternative to PAP therapy with low associated side effects and morbidity.
- New strategies are evolving to address individualized sleep apnea treatment options.

INTRODUCTION: AIRWAY AS A CULPRIT FOR SLEEP APNEA

Sleep apnea is a disease characterized by respiratory disturbances during sleep and associated with significant morbidity and mortality.[1] Obstructive sleep apnea (OSA) is the most common type of sleep apnea; however, it remains underdiagnosed and undertreated.[2] The underlying pathophysiology leading to OSA is often complex given that different phenotypes of OSA have been proposed. Given a wide range of disease severity, the treatment goal is to address the disease based on individual characteristics and needs.

The upper airway incorporates various rigid and collapsible structures that function in coordination to allow breathing, speech, and deglutition. It is thought that sleep-related changes in upper airway muscle tone is at least partially responsible for the development of OSA; however, both anatomic and nonanatomic factors likely contribute to airway obstruction.[3] For the past 4 decades, positive airway pressure (PAP) has been the mainstay of OSA treatment. Over the years, significant improvements in mask design and flow technology have been made to address issues related to PAP mask tolerance. Despite that, a large percentage of patients continue to struggle to adhere to long-term PAP therapy.[4,5] In order to address this unmet need, alternative treatments have been developed. These treatments include a variety of surgical

[a] Department of Otolaryngology–Head and Neck Surgery, Weill Cornell Medicine/NewYork-Presbyterian Hospital, 1300 York Avenue, New York, NY 10065, USA; [b] Departments of Medicine, Neurology and Genetic Medicine, Weill Cornell Medicine/NewYork-Presbyterian Hospital, 1300 York Avenue, New York, NY 10065, USA
* Corresponding author.
E-mail address: ack2003@med.cornell.edu

Clin Geriatr Med 37 (2021) 429–444
https://doi.org/10.1016/j.cger.2021.04.005
0749-0690/21/© 2021 Elsevier Inc. All rights reserved.

geriatric.theclinics.com

and nonsurgical approaches to improve airway patency during sleep, such as positional devices, oral appliances, upper airway surgery, and neurostimulation treatment. The last 3 approaches are discussed in this article.

ORAL APPLIANCES

The use of custom-made oral appliances, including mandibular advancement devices (MADs), may serve as a less invasive treatment option for OSA. The MADs consist of dual plates (superior and inferior) that are interconnected and often adjustable. They are often effective in opening the posterior pharyngeal space by displacing the mandible forward during sleep. By doing so, they also advance the base of tongue because it is inserted on the chin. There are various designs that provide customization to allow variable degrees of mandibular and tongue advancement, mouth opening, and movement. Custom-made adjustable MADs tend to have better outcomes and result in fewer side effects than over-the-counter boil-and-bite devices. Dentists specializing in sleep medicine are trained in evaluating patients with OSA for MADs to ensure they are appropriate candidates based on their facial anatomy and dental health.[6]

A different (non-MAD) oral appliance is the tongue-retaining device (TRD). These devices consist of plastic bulbs where the tongue is inserted. By using suction, the TRDs hold the tongue in a protruded position during sleep, which is kept inside the bulb. There are not many data on TRD effectiveness, and it can create tongue discomfort, dryness, and numbness, thus leading to poor adherence.[7]

MADs are considered a first-line therapy or alternative to PAP therapy in patients with mild-to-moderate OSA and second-line therapy for patients with severe OSA who have failed PAP therapy.[8] Prospective randomized controlled studies have shown efficacy of MAD in reduction of apnea-hypopnea index (AHI) and Epworth Sleepiness Scale (ESS) compared with no intervention.[9,10]

Both PAP and MAD are effective in reducing AHI and daytime sleepiness in patients with OSA. However, PAP was shown to have greater AHI reduction and to be more effective than MAD when treating more severe or more symptomatic OSA, and these devices were comparable in treating mild disease.[11–13] MAD has higher reported nightly compliance than PAP. Objective monitoring of MAD adherence has recently become available and it uses an embedded temperature sensor, which allows better compliance monitoring in clinical practice.[14]

During initial use of MADs, patients may experience excessive salivation, mouth dryness, tooth pain, gum irritation, headaches, and temporomandibular joint (TMJ) discomfort. These symptoms usually resolve within 2 months after therapy initiation.[15] A key issue with the use of MADs is the need for close monitoring with a dentist specializing in sleep medicine; the appliance may need to be replaced or adjusted over time with extended use. Persistent TMJ pain, loosening or shifting of the teeth, and occlusion changes are significant potential side effects of MAD usage and often an indication to discontinue treatment.[16,17]

Despite MADs being considered an alternative to PAP treatment, adjunctive use of both therapies can be considered in certain circumstances. Some patients who find oral appliances more socially acceptable and easier to use when traveling alternate between MAD and PAP use. In addition, combination therapy with MAD has a potential to improve PAP tolerance by creating more airway opening and reducing required pressure.

UPPER AIRWAY SURGERY

In 1974, Simmons and Hill[18] described daytime somnolence caused by chronic intermittent airway obstruction, which, when surgically corrected, resulted in disappearance of symptoms. This initial report described permanent tracheostomy in 1 case and correction on nasal septal deviation in the second case as surgical interventions that were able to manage airway obstruction during sleep.[18] Historically, surgical procedures for management of OSA involved site-specific reduction or repositioning of soft tissue or skeletal structures in order to increase upper airway dimensions. Procedures may include palatal surgery, tonsillectomy/adenoidectomy, hyoid suspension, tongue resection or suspension, genioglossus advancement, maxillomandibular advancement, and tracheostomy. These procedures can be performed as single-level procedures addressing 1 site of obstruction or as multilevel procedures combining surgery at multiple sites of obstruction. Even with the multilevel surgical approach, the success rates are variable and are associated with painful recovery and variable morbidity.

Nasal Surgery

Nasal breathing has been associated with airway stability during sleep, and nasal obstruction was shown to negatively affect airway collapsibility. Using a Starling resistor model, nasal obstruction increases upstream resistance, which creates negative pressure of the downstream airway (oropharynx and hypopharynx), resulting in higher collapsibility of already vulnerable structures.[19] Nasal breathing is advantageous given that it results in sensory stimulation that signals to increase airway muscle tone. In contrast, mouth breathing has been shown to increase airway resistance during sleep and is associated with retropalatal/retroglossal airway collapse.[20] Thus, evaluation of nasal breathing impediments during sleep and treatment of nasal obstruction are important in management of OSA.

When considering causes of nasal obstruction, attention should be paid to static and dynamic aspects of the problem. Nasal septal deviation, nasal framework, size of piriform aperture, nasal polyps, enlarged or pneumatized nasal turbinates, and adenoid hypertrophy are considered static causes of nasal obstruction and nasal valve collapse, whereas fluctuation of turbinate size, mucosal edema, inflammatory factors, body position, and fluid shifts are considered dynamic causes. Depending on the underlying cause of nasal obstruction, combination of medical and surgical treatment might be needed to achieve optimal nasal patency. Surgery to relieve nasal obstruction may include septoplasty, turbinate reduction, rhinoplasty, nasal valve repair, and endoscopic sinus surgery. Published meta-analyses show that isolated nasal surgery in patients with OSA improves nasal resistance, ESS score, and respiratory disturbance index,[21,22] and a more recent meta-analysis showed a slightly significant decrease in the AHI.[22]

Nasal obstruction is a common complaint among PAP users,[23] and higher nasal resistance was found to correlate with poor PAP therapy adherence.[24] Surgically enlarging nasal airways and decreasing nasal resistance is often considered in PAP nonadherent patients. A meta-analysis by Camacho and colleagues[25] showed that nasal surgery can reduce PAP pressure and increase adherence to PAP.

Palatal Surgery

Soft tissue surgery for sleep apnea is intended to increase the diameter of the airway and to reduce the size of the structures causing its obstruction. Uvulopalatopharyngoplasty (UPPP) has been the most commonly performed surgery for OSA.[26] The procedure was first introduced by Fujita and colleagues[27] and involved removal of redundant tissue of the soft palate and uvula in addition to tonsillectomy. This surgery targets obstruction at the velopharyngeal and oropharyngeal sites. In properly selected patients, it may be offered as a monotherapy or as part of multilevel surgery.

Multiple studies have assessed the UPPP success rate. Friedman and colleagues[28] have published on the outcomes based on palate position and tonsil size. Success rate was 80% in patients with large tonsils and palate position 1/2 (Friedman stage I). However, success rate in patients with small or no tonsils and palate position 3/4 was only 8%.[28] A meta-analysis of published randomized controlled studies on effectiveness of UPPP found that it was significantly more effective in reducing AHI and ESS compared with no treatment. Combined results from randomized controlled studies showed reduction of AHI from 35.4 events per hour to 17.9 events per hour in properly selected patients.[29,30]

Upper airway edema, postoperative bleeding and functional deficit of the soft palate are the main complications reported following UPPP.[31] Kezirian and colleagues[32] reported an overall complication rate of 1.3%. Lateral pharyngoplasty and expansion sphincteroplasty are some of the modifications that have been introduced to further improve outcomes of palatal surgery.[33,34] Pang and colleagues[35] reported that patients who underwent expansion palatoplasty achieved an 82% success rate versus patients treated with traditional UPPP, who had a 68% success rate. Despite the variable reported success rates of UPPP in treating OSA, patients who underwent surgery consistently report improved quality of life.[36]

Laser-assisted uvuloplasty (LAUP) was introduced as an in-office palatal procedure performed under local anesthesia to treat snoring and OSA.[37] Early meta-analysis of LAUP concluded that, because of the paucity of long-term data, the procedure should not be recommended for treatment of OSA.[38] A more recent study showed a success rate of 23%, cure rate of 8%, and worsening of the AHI among 44% of patients.[39] Globus sensation and velopharyngeal insufficiency are significant complications associated with the procedure.[40]

Base of Tongue and Hypopharyngeal Surgery

The nature of airway obstruction is variable in individual patients with OSA, and airway collapse during sleep often occurs on multiple anatomic levels. The palate is the most common site of airway obstruction, and the combination of palatal and base of tongue is the most frequently observed site of multilevel collapse.[41]

Various techniques have been developed for base of tongue reduction with the goal of alleviating airway obstruction during sleep. Radiofrequency ablation (RFA) delivers energy to the tongue base tissues at multiple zones using an electrode probe. This energy creates tissue inflammation and subsequent scarring leading to volume reduction.[42] Midline glossectomy was introduced in 1991[43] and, since then, different techniques have been used to excise the base of tongue[44,45] or submucosally reduce tongue tissue with radiofrequency.[46] With the introduction of robotic technology, Vicini and colleagues[47] showed that transoral robotic surgery (TORS) is an effective treatment of OSA associated with tongue base airway obstruction. The procedure involves bilateral lingual tonsillectomy or base of tongue and epiglottis reduction using robotic technology. In properly selected patients, the success rate of TORS has been shown to be 76.6%.[48] Bleeding, dysphagia, and hypogeusia are the most commonly reported complications. Compared with other base of tongue reduction techniques, TORS provides better visualization during surgery, allows more controlled and consistent removal of lingual tissue, and leads to better results. However, it is associated with a higher rate of complications and significant costs.[49]

Hyoid surgery has been introduced to further expand the hypopharyngeal airway and decrease obstruction at the tongue base by providing anterior movement of the hyoid complex. The original technique involved inferior hyoid myotomy and suspension of the hyoid to the mandible,[50] which was later modified to hyoidthyroidopexy, which brought the hyoid bone anteroinferiorly by fixing it to the thyroid cartilage.[51] A systematic review concluded that current literature on the subject lacks high-quality evidence, but isolated hyoid surgery may reduce OSA severity.[52]

Skeletal Surgery

Anterior movement of the mandible to improve hypopharyngeal obstruction in patients with OSA was reported by Powel and colleagues[53] in 1983. At present, maxillomandibular advancement (MMA) offers multilevel airway enlargement by advancement of both the maxilla and the mandible. MMA is a surgical option offered to patients with OSA who are unable to tolerate PAP or who have failed other surgical interventions. As a result of the multilevel effect on the airway, MMA is considered an effective OSA treatment, with surgical success rate of 85.5% and cure rate of 38.5%. Preoperative AHI less than 60 events per hour is associated with a higher rate of surgical cure, and patients with higher preoperative AHI had more significant changes in outcomes measures.[54] Meta-analysis of the long-term results of MMA showed that patients who were treated with MMA maintained improvements in AHI and ESS, and had the lowest oxygen saturation; however, AHI increased over the very long term.[55]

MMA is an invasive procedure that is associated with adverse events such as pain, swelling, malocclusion, poor cosmetic result, facial numbness, tingling, jaw stiffness, postsurgical relapse of advancement, bleeding, local infection, and extrusion of hardware. Transient anesthesia of the lower lip, chin, and cheek is seen in all patients in the immediate postoperative period and resolves between 6 and 12 months in 87% of patients.[56] It is advisable to select a specialized and experienced team for decision making and care of patients considering MMA surgery.

HYPOGLOSSAL NERVE STIMULATION

Given that nonanatomic causes of OSA include an inadequate neuromuscular response of the upper airway dilator muscles during sleep,[57] research focusing on submental and submaxillary transcutaneous stimulation as a treatment of airway obstruction during sleep started to develop in the late 1990s.[58,59] Over the years, this concept was further refined and changed its focus from muscle-directed approaches to the nerves, which showed improved tolerance and lower potential for adverse effects.[60]

In animal models, an increase in the upper airway dimension was found in response to hypoglossal nerve stimulation (HGNS).[61–65] In 2001, Schwartz and colleagues[66] showed that unilateral HGNS decreased severity of OSA in 8 patients with no adverse effects to stimulation. Research in this field escalated and companies started to develop their own devices for HGNS in patients with OSA. In 2014, as a result of successful clinical trials, the US Food and Drug Administration (FDA) approved a hypoglossal nerve electrical stimulation device (manufactured by Inspire Medical Systems, Maple Grove, MN) for treatment of OSA in patients that failed to respond to PAP.[67]

The Stimulation Therapy for Apnea Reduction (STAR) trial data showed a 68% reduction in AHI from a baseline of 29.3 to 9.0 events per hour after 12 months of HGNS therapy. A similar reduction was seen in oxygen desaturation index, from 25.4 to 7.4 events per hour in this same trial. Therapeutic efficacy of HGNS was achieved in 66% of the patients who met the inclusion criteria.[67] Subjective measures, including the ESS and Functional Outcomes of Sleep Questionnaire (FOSQ) scores, showed clinically significant improvement from baseline. Longer-term patient follow-up of the prospective phase III STAR trial showed persistent reduction in AHI with the therapy use.[67-72] Posttrial single-center[73,74] and multicenter studies[75,76] have shown the effectiveness of HGNS in clinical practice. A follow-up to the STAR trial, the multicenter ADHERE (Adherence and Outcome of Upper Airway Stimulation for OSA International Registry), gathers data from patients treated with HGNS with respect to demographics, surgical outcomes, complications, quality of life, and patient-reported outcomes. The ADHERE data from the first 301 patients reported average therapy compliance of 6.5 hours per night and an AHI reduction from a baseline of 35.6 to 10.2 events per hour. As for patient-reported response to therapy, 90% of patients reported a better experience than continuous positive airway pressure (CPAP); 96% would choose the procedure again; 94% would recommend the procedure to a friend or family member; and, overall, 92% were satisfied with therapy.[77]

More recent ADHERE reports found a positive association between older age and therapy success. There is a trend toward women having increased odds of therapeutic success.[78,79] This report similarly showed high patient therapy satisfaction and low rate of adverse events.

Based on the outcomes of the STAR clinical trial and FDA recommendations, HGNS therapy is indicated for adult patients 18 years of age and older with moderate to severe OSA with an AHI of at least 15 but no more than 65 events per hour, of which less than 25% are central/mixed, who have failed or cannot tolerate PAP treatment, and who do not have complete concentric collapse (CCC) at the soft palate level on drug-induced sleep endoscopy (DISE), as shown in **Fig. 1.**

Before the STAR trial, Vanderveken and colleagues[80] studied the role of DISE as a patient selection tool for HGNS. The study reported on 21 patients who underwent DISE and HGNS implant placement and found a statistically significant AHI reduction difference between patients with and without CCC, which led to the conclusion that absence of CCC can predict the success rate of HGNS. For body mass index (BMI), there are no definitive FDA restrictions. However, the STAR trial only included patients with BMI less than 32 kg/m²,[67] and patients with BMI less than 35 kg/m² had greater AHI reduction with HGNS.[81] Data from the most recent ADHERE publications suggested inverse association of BMI and HGNS therapy effectiveness.[78,79] Pooled analysis of 4 studies on outcomes of HGNS that combined data for 584 patients revealed greater reduction in AHI associated with a higher preoperative AHI, older patient age, and lower BMI.[82] Another study found no difference in HGNS therapy success rate between groups with BMI greater than 32 kg/m² and BMI less than 32 kg/m².[83]

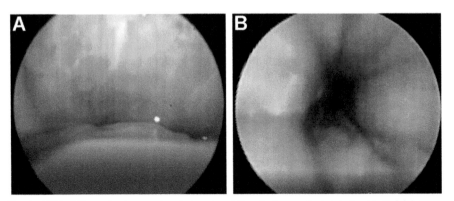

Fig. 1. DISE at the velopharynx level showing (*A*) anterior-posterior collapse and (*B*) CCC.

The current FDA-approved HGNS device is shown in **Fig. 2** and consists of 3 parts: a respiratory sensor lead, an implantable pulse generator, and a nerve stimulation electrode cuff. The device is implanted subcutaneously unilaterally, preferably on the right side during an outpatient procedure under general anesthesia by a trained surgeon.[84]

The hypoglossal nerve, or cranial nerve XII, innervates extrinsic and intrinsic tongue muscles. The main trunk of the hypoglossal nerve divides into lateral and medial branches, as shown in **Fig. 3**. The lateral branch innervates the extrinsic retrusor (styloglossus, hyoglossus) muscles and the medial branches innervate the extrinsic protrusor (genioglossus) and intrinsic muscles of the tongue responsible for stiffening and shape changes.[85] Cervical spinal nerve 1 (C1) innervates the geniohyoid muscle and, with stimulation, it moves the hyoid bone anteriorly allowing increased airway opening.[86] The goal of the HGNS is to have bilateral forward or rightward protrusion of the tongue.[87] Thus, precise placement of the neurostimulation cuff on the protrusor or medial branches of the hypoglossal nerve is essential for improved clinical outcomes. HGNS therapy provides multilevel airway opening without altering airway anatomy[88] and it can be programmed to optimize individual therapy effects. This procedure carries significantly lower complication rates, is associated with minimal postoperative discomfort, and has much shorter recovery time compared with other surgeries for OSA.[89]

Small studies in special populations, such as patients with Down syndrome with severe OSA, have shown HGNS to be effective, with adequate compliance, improved quality of sleep, and significant AHI reduction.[90] Although the HGNS is approved for adult patients with OSA, safety of therapy was also reported in a small series of adolescent patients with Down syndrome.[91]

In patients that have residual disease after implantation, combination therapy could be considered. Reports have shown improved outcomes when HGNS therapy was

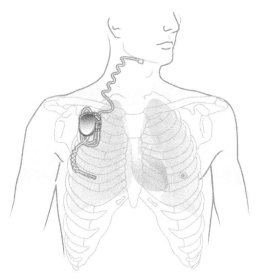

Fig. 2. Inspire hypoglossal nerve stimulation implant. The respiratory sensor is implanted in the intercoastal space, the implantable pulse generator is implanted in the upper chest, and the stimulator cuff is connected to the hypoglossal nerve subcutaneously. (*Courtesy of* Inspire Medical Systems, Inc.)

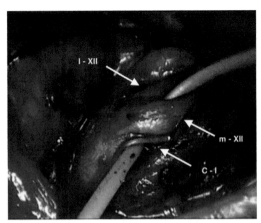

Fig. 3. Hypoglossal nerve stimulation lead placement by identification of the branches: medial branches (m-XII) are separated from the lateral branches (l-XII) with a vascular loop in blue. The stimulation cuff is placed to include m-XII and the C-1 nerve, which innervates the geniohyoid muscle. The m-XII innervates genioglossus muscles and l-XII innervates styloglossus and hyoglossus.

combined with a chin strap,[92] oral appliance,[93] positional therapy,[94] and uvulopalatopharyngoplasty.[95]

When taking into consideration the societal costs of untreated sleep apnea, HGNS therapy was found to be a cost-effective treatment option for patients with moderate to severe sleep apnea that experienced failure of CPAP treatment.[96]

NEUROSTIMULATION DEVICE FOR CENTRAL SLEEP APNEA

Central sleep apnea (CSA) is more commonly seen in patients with underlying cardiac or neurologic comorbidities. In patients with heart failure, CSA was shown to be an independent risk factor for cardiac-related hospital readmissions at 6 months.[97] Newly diagnosed CSA during a hospital admission for heart failure is independently associated with postdischarge mortality.[98] At present, there are limited effective treatment options for patients with CSA. Most clinical evidence for CSA treatment is based on small short-term trials. Similarly to OSA, PAP is considered a standard initial treatment modality for patients with CSA. Use of continuous PAP for treatment of CSA was effective in improving central apneas, oxygen saturation, ejection fraction, and tolerance to physical activity, but it failed to show survival benefit.[99] Controversial data on the use of adaptive servoventilation have been described, particularly when empirically prescribed in patients with moderate to severe CSA, symptomatic heart failure, and reduced left ventricular ejection fraction of less than 45%.[100,101]

In October 2017, the FDA approved the remedē System (Respicardia, Minnetonka, MN) implantable device to treat moderate to severe CSA. The remedē system consists of an implantable pulse generator and a transvenous lead for unilateral stimulation of the phrenic nerve. The remedē system is programmed to deliver electrical impulses to the phrenic nerve throughout the night, causing the diaphragm to contract, triggering a breath. The randomized controlled remedē System Pivotal Trial enrolled 151 patients with CSA. A greater proportion of patients treated with phrenic nerve stimulation experienced greater than 50% reduction in the AHI after 6 months compared with the control. Sixty-four percent of patients in the trial had CSA and associated heart failure.[102]

Effectiveness of the therapy was maintained at 12 months. The sustained benefit was present across all secondary sleep indices, measures of sleep quality, and patient-reported outcomes.[103]

DEVICES UNDER RESEARCH

Other neurostimulation systems for OSA are currently being investigated. The aurora6000 system (LivaNova, London, United Kingdom) provides continuous stimulation of the hypoglossal nerve without respiratory synchronization. In contrast with the Inspire system, a cuff with 6 independent contact electrodes is placed on the main trunk of the hypoglossal nerve for stimulation. The targeted hypoglossal neurostimulation (THN) cycles between contact electrodes and reduces OSA severity by maintaining the tone of the tongue muscles. A multicenter cohort study on THN therapy evaluated the effectiveness of the device in 46 patients. At 6 months after implantation, the mean AHI reduction from a baseline of 34.9 ± 22.5 (mean $\pm$ SD) to 25.4 ± 23.1 events per hour.[104] In the responder group, the AHI was reduced from 32.1 ± 14.5 (mean $\pm$ SD) to 11.3 ± 7.4 events per hour. Further analysis suggested that the severity of the disease and selection criteria were potential predictors of the therapeutic response, including obesity. Further trials are ongoing to help establish therapy outcomes and guide patient selection.

Genio Implantable Stimulator system (Nyxoah SA, Mont-St-Guibert, Belgium) is another neurostimulation system that is under clinical trial investigation. This system consists of 2 sets of paired stimulating electrodes and a receiving antenna. It is implanted under the chin over both genioglossus muscles. The paddle of the electrodes is placed in contact with the medial branches of hypoglossal nerve bilaterally. The system does not contain a battery; it uses an external adhesive device activation unit with wireless transmission and the stimulation is not synchronized with respiration. The patient places the adhesive patch under the chin and removes it on awakening.[105] The activation unit holds patient-specific stimulation parameters that are programmed during wake and attended titration studies. Recently published data on the outcomes of 22 patients showed average AHI decreases from 23.7 ± 12.2 (mean $\pm$ SD) to 12.9 ± 10.1 events per hour and significant improvement of ESS, FOSQ, snoring, and sleep efficiency after 6 months of device use. No device-related serious adverse events were observed.[106,107]

Given the nature of the electrical stimulation, careful consideration must be given in case patients require routine MRI studies because of safety concerns when using any of the neurostimulator devices mentioned earlier.

FUTURE DIRECTION

Several non-PAP options for managing OSA are currently available. Targeted and individualized treatment should be considered in order to improve effectiveness and overall adherence.[57] These options include the use of oral appliances, positional restriction, and upper airway surgical procedures, including the implantation of neurostimulators, which can be an effective treatment of sleep apnea in properly selected patients. Furthermore, combination of therapies should be considered in case of residual disease. Special consideration should also be given to behavioral interventions that could help attenuate sleep apnea, including avoidance of sedatives and alcoholic beverages, and weight reduction, which are beyond the scope of this report. In summary, a comprehensive and personalized approach should be the cornerstone for managing sleep apnea, with full consideration of the therapeutic options currently available.

CLINICS CARE POINTS

- The management of Obstructive Sleep Apnea (OSA) often requires a personalized approach to determine the best therapy for each individual patient.
- Non-PAP approaches should be considered when patients fail to tolerate PAP use.
- Hypoglossal nerve stimulation is an effective approach to reduce the severity of OSA in a selected group of patients.

DISCLOSURE

Research support: Dr Suurna received honoraria from Inspire Medical Systems.

REFERENCES

1. Dempsey JA, Veasey SC, Morgan BJ, et al. Pathophysiology of sleep apnea [published correction appears in Physiol Rev.2010 Apr;90(2):797-8. Physiol Rev 2010;90(1):47–112.
2. Frost & Sullivan. Hidden health crisis costing America billions. Underdiagnosing and undertreating obstructive sleep apnea draining healthcare system. American Academy of Sleep Medicine; 2016. Available at: https://aasm.org/resources/pdf/sleep-apnea-economic-crisis.pdf.
3. Remmers JE, deGroot WJ, Sauerland EK, et al. Pathogenesis of upper airway occlusion during sleep. J Appl Physiol Respir Environ Exerc Physiol 1978; 44(6):931–8.
4. Rotenberg BW, Murariu D, Pang KP. Trends in CPAP adherence over twenty years of data collection: a flattened curve. J Otolaryngol Head Neck Surg 2016;45:43.
5. Sawyer AM, Gooneratne NS, Marcus CL, et al. A systematic review of CPAP adherence across age groups: clinical and empiric insights for developing CPAP adherence interventions. Sleep Med Rev 2011;15(6):343–56.
6. Hoffstein V. Review of oral appliances for treatment of sleep-disordered breathing. Sleep Breath 2007;11(1):1–22.
7. Deane SA, Cistulli PA, Ng AT, et al. Comparison of mandibular advancement splint and tongue stabilizing device in obstructive sleep apnea: a randomized controlled trial. Sleep 2009;32(5):648–53.
8. Kushida CA, Littner MR, Morgenthaler T, et al. Practice parameters for the indications for polysomnography and related procedures: an update for 2005. Sleep 2005;28(4):499–521.
9. Blanco J, Zamarron C, Abeleira Pazos MT, et al. Prospective evaluation of an oral appliance in the treatment of obstructive sleep apnea syndrome. Sleep Breath 2005;9:20–5.
10. Petri N, Svanholt P, Solow B, et al. Mandibular advancement appliance for obstructive sleep apnoea: results of a randomised placebo controlled trial using parallel group design. J Sleep Res 2008;17:221–9.
11. Bratton DJ, Gaisl T, Schlatzer C, et al. Comparison of the effects of continuous positive airway pressure and mandibular advancement devices on sleepiness in patients with obstructive sleep apnoea: a network meta-analysis. Lancet Respir Med 2015;3:869–78.
12. Sharples LD, Clutterbuck-James AL, Glover MJ, et al. Meta-analysis of randomised controlled trials of oral mandibular advancement devices and continuous

positive airway pressure for obstructive sleep apnoea-hypopnoea. Sleep Med Rev 2016;27:108–24.

13. Engleman HM, McDonald JP, Graham D, et al. Randomized crossover trial of two treatments for sleep apnea/hypopnea syndrome: continuous positive airway pressure and mandibular repositioning splint. Am J Respir Crit Care Med 2002; 166(6):855–9.

14. Sutherland K, Vanderveken OM, Tsuda H, et al. Oral appliance treatment for obstructive sleep apnea: an update. J Clin Sleep Med 2014;10:215–27.

15. Giannasi LC, Almeida FR, Magini M, et al. Systematic assessment of the impact of oral appliance therapy on the temporomandibular joint during treatment of obstructive sleep apnea: long-term evaluation. Sleep Breath 2009;13:375–81.

16. de Almeida FR, Lowe AA, Tsuiki S, et al. Long-term compliance and side effects of oral appliances used for the treatment of snoring and obstructive sleep apnea syndrome. J Clin Sleep Med 2005;1:143–52.

17. El-Solh AA, Moitheennazima B, Akinnusi ME, et al. Combined oral appliance and positive airway pressure therapy for obstructive sleep apnea: a pilot study. Sleep Breath 2011;15(2):203–8.

18. Simmons FB, Hill MW. Hypersomnia caused by upper airway obstructions: a new syndrome in otolaryngology. Ann Otol Rhinol Laryngol 1974;83(5):670–3.

19. Le TB, Moghaddam MG, Woodson BT, et al. Airflow limitation in a collapsible model of the human pharynx: physical mechanisms studied with fluid-structure interaction simulations and experiments. Physiol Rep 2019;7:1–15.

20. Fitzpatrick MF, McLean H, Urton AM, et al. Effect of nasal or oral breathing route on upper airway resistance during sleep. Eur Respir J 2003;22(5):827–32.

21. Ishii L, Roxbury C, Godoy A, et al. Does nasal surgery improve OSA in patients with nasal obstruction and OSA? A meta-analysis. Otolaryngol Head Neck Surg 2015;153(3):326–33.

22. Wu J, Zhao G, Li Y, et al. Apnea-hypopnea index decreased significantly after nasal surgery for obstructive sleep apnea: a meta-analysis. Medicine (Baltimore) 2017;96(5):e6008.

23. Hoffstein V, Viner S, Mateika S, et al. Treatment of obstructive sleep apnea with nasal continuous positive airway pressure. Patient compliance, perception of benefits, and side effects. Am Rev Respir Dis 1992;145(4 Pt 1):841–5.

24. Sugiura T, Noda A, Nakata S, et al. Influence of nasal resistance on initial acceptance of continuous positive airway pressure in treatment for obstructive sleep apnea syndrome. Respiration 2007;74(1):56–60.

25. Camacho M, Riaz M, Capasso R, et al. The effect of nasal surgery on continuous positive airway pressure device use and therapeutic treatment pressures: a systematic review and meta-analysis. Sleep 2015;38(2):279–86.

26. Kezirian EJ, Maselli J, Vittinghoff E, et al. Obstructive sleep apnea surgery practice patterns in the United States: 2000 to 2006. Otolaryngol Head Neck Surg 2010;143(3):441–7.

27. Fujita S, Conway W, Zorick F, et al. Surgical correction of anatomic abnormalities in obstructive sleep apnea syndrome: uvulopalatopharyngoplasty. Otolaryngol Head Neck Surg 1981;89:923–34.

28. Friedman M, Ibrahim H, Joseph NJ. Staging of obstructive sleep apnea/hypopnea syndrome: a guide to appropriate treatment. The Laryngoscope 2004; 114(3):454–9.

29. Browaldh N, Bring J, Friberg D. SKUP 3 RCT; continuous study: changes in sleepiness and quality of life after modified UPPP. Laryngoscope 2016;126(6): 1484–91.

30. Sommer UJ, Heiser C, Gahleitner C, et al. Tonsillectomy with uvulopalatopharyngoplasty in obstructive sleep apnea. Dtsch Arztebl Int 2016;113(1–02):1–8.

31. Stuck BA, Ravesloot MJ, Eschenhagen T, et al. Uvulopalatopharyngoplasty with or without tonsillectomy in the treatment of adult obstructive sleep apnea–A systematic review. Sleep Med 2018;50:152–65.

32. Kezirian EJ, Weaver EM, Yueh B, et al. Risk factors for serious complication after uvulopalatopharyngoplasty. Arch Otolaryngol Head Neck Surg 2006;132(10): 1091–8.

33. Cahali MB. Lateral pharyngoplasty: a new treatment for obstructive sleep apnea hypopnea syndrome. Laryngoscope 2003;113(11):1961–8.

34. Woodson B, Sitton M, Jacobowitz O. Expansion sphincter pharyngoplasty and palatal advancement pharyngoplasty: airway evaluation and surgical techniques. Oper Tech Otolaryngol 2012;23(1):3–10.

35. Pang KP, Woodson BT. Expansion sphincter pharyngoplasty: a new technique for the treatment of obstructive sleep apnea. Otolaryngol Head Neck Surg 2007;137:110–4.

36. Weaver EM, Woodson BT, Yueh B, et al. Studying Life Effects & Effectiveness of Palatopharyngoplasty (SLEEP) study: subjective outcomes of isolated uvulopalatopharyngoplasty. Otolaryngol Head Neck Surg 2011;144(4):623–31.

37. Kamami YV. Outpatient treatment of sleep apnea syndrome with CO_2 laser, LAUP: laser-assisted UPPP results on 46 patients. J Clin Laser Med Surg 1994;12(4):215–9.

38. Verse T, Pirsig W. Metaanalyse zur laserassistierten Uvulopalatopharyngoplastik. Was ist bisher klinisch relevant? [Meta-analysis of laser-assisted uvulopalatopharyngoplasty. What is clinically relevant up to now?]. Laryngorhinootologie 2000;79(5):273–84.

39. Camacho M, Nesbitt NB, Lambert E, et al. Laser-assisted uvulopalatoplasty for obstructive sleep apnea: a systematic review and meta-analysis. Sleep 2017; 40(3):10.

40. Wischhusen J, Qureshi U, Camacho M. Laser-assisted uvulopalatoplasty (LAUP) complications and side effects: a systematic review. Nat Sci Sleep 2019;11:59–67.

41. Vroegop AV, Vanderveken OM, Boudewyns AN, et al. Drug-induced sleep endoscopy in sleep-disordered breathing: report on 1,249 cases. Laryngoscope 2014;124(3):797–802.

42. Powell NB, Riley RW, Guilleminault C. Radiofrequency tongue base reduction in sleep-disordered breathing: a pilot study. Otolaryngol Head Neck Surg 1999; 120(5):656–64.

43. Dorrity J, Wirtz N, Froymovich O, et al. Genioglossal advancement, hyoid suspension, tongue base radiofrequency, and endoscopic partial midline glossectomy for obstructive sleep apnea. Otolaryngol Clin North Am 2016;49(6): 1399–414.

44. Fujita S, Woodson BT, Clark JL, et al. Laser midline glossectomy as a treatment for obstructive sleep apnea. Laryngoscope 1991;101(8):805–9.

45. Woodson BT, Fujita S. Clinical experience with lingualplasty as part of the treatment of severe obstructive sleep apnea. Otolaryngol Head Neck Surg 1992; 107(1):40–8.

46. Robinson S, Lewis R, Norton A, et al. Ultrasound-guided radiofrequency submucosal tongue-base excision for sleep apnoea: a preliminary report. Clin Otolaryngol Allied Sci 2003;28(4):341–5.

47. Vicini C, Dallan I, Canzi P, et al. Transoral robotic tongue base resection in obstructive sleep apnoea-hypopnoea syndrome: a preliminary report. ORL J Otorhinolaryngol Relat Spec 2010;72(1):22–7.

48. Vicini C, Montevecchi F, Gobbi R, et al. Transoral robotic surgery for obstructive sleep apnea syndrome: principles and technique. World J Otorhinolaryngol Head Neck Surg 2017;3(2):97–100.

49. Cammaroto G, Montevecchi F, D'Agostino G, et al. Tongue reduction for OSAHS: TORSs vs coblations, Technologies vs techniques, apples vs oranges. Eur Arch Otorhinolaryngol 2017;274(2):637–45.

50. Riley R, Guilleminault C, Powell N, et al. Mandibular osteotomy and hyoid bone advancement for obstructive sleep apnea: a case report. Sleep 1984;7:79–82.

51. Riley RW, Powell NB, Guilleminault C. Obstructive sleep apnea and the hyoid: a revised surgical procedure. Otolaryngol Head Neck Surg 1994;111:717–21.

52. Song SA, Wei JM, Buttram J, et al. Hyoid surgery alone for obstructive sleep apnea: a systematic review and meta-analysis. Laryngoscope 2016;126(7): 1702–8.

53. Powell NB, Guilleminault C, Riley RW. Mandibular advancement and obstructive sleep apnea syndrome. Bull Eur Physiopathol Respir 1983;19:607–10.

54. Zaghi S, Holty JE, Certal V, et al. Maxillomandibular advancement for treatment of obstructive sleep apnea: a meta-analysis. JAMA Otolaryngol Head Neck Surg 2016;142(1):58–66.

55. Camacho M, Noller MW, Del Do M, et al. Long-term results for maxillomandibular advancement to treat obstructive sleep apnea: a meta-analysis. Otolaryngol Head Neck Surg 2019;160(4):580–93.

56. Li KK, Powell NB, Riley RW, et al. Long-term results of maxillomandibular advancement surgery. Sleep Breath 2000;4(3):137–40.

57. Eckert DJ, White DP, Jordan AS, et al. Defining phenotypic causes of obstructive sleep apnea. Identification of novel therapeutic targets. Am J Respir Crit Care Med 2013;188(8):996–1004.

58. Miki H, Hida W, Chonan T, et al. Effects of submental electrical stimulation during sleep on upper airway patency in patients with obstructive sleep apnea. Am Rev Respir Dis 1989;140(5):1285–9.

59. Hida W, Okabe S, Miki H, et al. Submental stimulation and supraglottic resistance during mouth breathing. Respir Physiol 1995;101(1):79–85.

60. Guilleminault C, Powell N, Bowman B, et al. The effect of electrical stimulation on obstructive sleep apnea syndrome. Chest 1995;107(1):67–73.

61. Schwartz AR, Thut DC, Russ B, et al. Effect of electrical stimulation of the hypoglossal nerve on airflow mechanics in the isolated upper airway. Am Rev Respir Dis 1993;147:1144–50.

62. Oliven A, Odeh M, Schnall RP. Improved upper airway patency elicited by electrical stimulation of the hypoglosssus nerves. Respiration 1996;63:213–6.

63. Eisele DW, Schwartz AR, Hari A, et al. The effects of selective nerve stimulation on upper airflow mechanics. Arch Otolaryngol Head Neck Surg 1995;121: 1361–4.

64. Bishara H, Odeh M, Schnall RP, et al. Electrically-activated dilator muscles reduce pharyngeal resistance in anaesthetized dogs with upper airway obstruction. Eur Respir J 1995;8:1537–42.

65. Goding GS, Eisele DW, Testerman R, et al. Relief of upper airway obstruction with hypoglossal nerve stimulation in the canine. Laryngoscope 1998;108: 162–9.

66. Schwartz AR, Benett ML, Smith PL, et al. Therapeutic electrical stimulation of the hypoglossal nerve in obstructive sleep apnea. Arch Otolaryngol Head Neck Surg 2001;127:1216–23.

67. Strollo PJ, Soose RJ, Maurer JT, et al. Upper-airway stimulation for obstructive sleep apnea. N Engl J Med 2014;370:139–49.

68. Strollo PJ, Gillespie MB, Soose RJ, et al. Upper airway stimulation for obstructive sleep apnea: durability of the treatment effect at 18 months. Sleep 2015;38(10): 1593–8.

69. Soose RJ, Woodson BT, Gillespie MB, et al. Upper airway stimulation for obstructive sleep apnea: self-reported outcomes at 24 months. J Clin Sleep Med 2016;12(1):43–8.

70. Woodson BT, Soose RJ, Gillespie MB, et al. Three-year outcomes of cranial nerve stimulation for obstructive sleep apnea: the STAR trial. Otolaryngol Head Neck Surg 2016;154(1):181–8.

71. Gillespie MB, Soose RJ, Woodson BT, et al. Upper airway stimulation for obstructive sleep apnea: patient-reported outcomes after 48 months of follow-up. Otolaryngol Head Neck Surg 2017;156(4):765–71.

72. Woodson BT, Strohl KP, Soose RJ, et al. Upper airway stimulation for obstructive sleep apnea: 5-year outcomes. Otolaryngol Head Neck Surg 2018;159(1): 194–202.

73. Heiser C, Knopf A, Bas M, et al. Selective upper airway stimulation for obstructive sleep apnea: a single center clinical experience. Eur Arch Otorhinolaryngol 2017;274(3):1727–34.

74. Kent DT, Lee JJ, Strollo PJ Jr, et al. Upper airway stimulation for OSA: early adherence and outcome results of one center. Otolaryngol Head Neck Surg 2016 Jul;155(1):188–93.

75. Steffen A, Sommer JU, Hofauer B, et al. Outcome after one year of upper airway stimulation for obstructive sleep apnea in a multicenter German post-market study. Laryngoscope 2017;128(2):509–15.

76. Huntley C, Kaffenberger T, Doghramji K, et al. Upper airway stimulation for treatment of obstructive sleep apnea: an evaluation and comparison of outcomes at two academic centers. J Clin Sleep Med 2017;13(9):1075–9.

77. Boon M, Huntley C, Steffen A, et al. Upper airway stimulation for obstructive sleep apnea: results from the ADHERE registry. Otolaryngol Head Neck Surg 2018;159(2):379–85.

78. Heiser C, Steffen A, Boon M, et al. Post-approval upper airway stimulation predictors of treatment effectiveness in the ADHERE registry. Eur Respir J 2019; 53(1):1801405.

79. Thaler E, Schwab R, Maurer J, et al. Results of the ADHERE upper airway stimulation registry and predictors of therapy efficacy. Laryngoscope 2020;130(5): 1333–8.

80. Vanderveken OM, Maurer JT, Hohenhorst W, et al. Evaluation of drug-induced sleep endoscopy as a patient selection tool for implanted upper airway stimulation for obstructive sleep apnea. J Clin Sleep Med 2013;9(5):433–8.

81. Kezirian EJ, Goding GS Jr, Malhotra A, et al. Hypoglossal nerve stimulation improves obstructive sleep apnea: 12-month outcomes. J Sleep Res 2014;23(1): 77–83.

82. Kent DT, Carden KA, Wang L, et al. Evaluation of hypoglossal nerve stimulation treatment in obstructive sleep apnea. JAMA Otolaryngol Head Neck Surg 2019; 145(11):1044–52.

83. Huntley C, Steffen A, Doghramji K, et al. Upper airway stimulation in patients with obstructive sleep apnea and an elevated body mass index: a multi-institutional review. Laryngoscope 2018;128(10):2425–8.

84. Heiser C, Thaler E, Boon M, et al. Updates of operative techniques for upper airway stimulation. Laryngoscope 2016;126(Suppl 7):S12–6.

85. Mu L, Sanders I. Human tongue neuroanatomy: nerve supply and motor end-plates. Clin Anat 2010;23(7):777–91.

86. Elshebiny T, Venkat D, Strohl K, et al. Hyoid arch displacement with hypoglossal nerve stimulation. Am J Respir Crit Care Med 2017;196(6):790–2.

87. Heiser C, Maurer JT, Steffen A. Functional outcome of tongue motions with selective hypoglossal nerve stimulation in patients with obstructive sleep apnea. Sleep Breath 2016;20:553–60.

88. Safiruddin F, Vanderveken OM, de Vries N, et al. Effect of upper-airway stimulation for obstructive sleep apnoea on airway dimensions. Eur Respir J 2015; 45(1):129–38.

89. Murphey AW, Baker AB, Soose RJ, et al. Upper airway stimulation for obstructive sleep apnea: the surgical learning curve. Laryngoscope 2016;126(2):501–6.

90. Li C, Boon M, Ishman SL, et al. Hypoglossal nerve stimulation in three adults with down syndrome and severe obstructive sleep apnea. Laryngoscope 2019;129(11):E402–6.

91. Diercks GR, Wentland C, Keamy D, et al. Hypoglossal nerve stimulation in adolescents with down syndrome and obstructive apnea. JAMA Otolaryngol Head Neck Surg 2017;44(1):E1–6.

92. Ramaswamy AT, Li C, Suurna MV. A case of hypoglossal nerve stimulator-resistant obstructive sleep apnea cured with the addition of a chin strap. Laryngoscope 2018;128(7):1727–9.

93. Lee JJ, Sahu N, Rogers R, et al. Severe obstructive sleep apnea treated with combination hypoglossal nerve stimulation and oral appliance therapy. J Dental Sleep Med 2015;2(4):185–6.

94. Steffen A, Hartmann JT, König IR, et al. Evaluation of body position in upper airway stimulation for obstructive sleep apnea-is continuous voltage sufficient enough? Sleep Breath 2018;22(4):1207–12.

95. Steffen A, Abrams N, Suurna MV, et al. Upper-Airway-Stimulation before, after or without uvulopalatopharyngoplasty - a two-year perspective. Laryngoscope 2019;129:514–8.

96. Pietzsch JB, Liu S, Garner AM, et al. Long-term cost-effectiveness of upper airway stimulation for the treatment of obstructive sleep apnea: a model-based projection based on the STAR trial. Sleep 2015;38(5):735–44.

97. Khayat R, Abraham W, Patt B, et al. Central sleep apnea is a predictor of cardiac readmission in hospitalized patients with systolic heart failure. J Card Fail 2012; 18(7):534–40.

98. Khayat R, Jarjoura D, Porter K, et al. Sleep disordered breathing and post-discharge mortality in patients with acute heart failure. Eur Heart J 2015; 36(23):1463–9.

99. Bradley TD, Logan AG, Kimoff RJ, et al. Continuous positive airway pressure for central sleep apnea and heart failure. N Engl J Med 2005;353(19):2025–33.

100. Cowie MR, Woehrle H, Wegscheider K, et al. Adaptive servo-ventilation for central sleep apnea in systolic heart failure. N Engl J Med 2015;373:1095–105.

101. Aurora RN, Bista SR, Casey KR, et al. Updated adaptive servo-ventilation recommendations for the 2012 AASM Guideline: "the treatment of central sleep

apnea syndromes in adults: practice parameters with an evidence-based literature review and meta-analyses". J Clin Sleep Med 2016;12:757–61.

102. Costanzo MR, Ponikowski P, Javaheri S, et al. Transvenous neurostimulation for central sleep apnoea: a randomised controlled trial. Lancet 2016;388:974–82.

103. Costanzo MR, Ponikowski P, Javaheri S, et al. Sustained 12 month benefit of phrenic nerve stimulation for central sleep apnea. Am J Cardiol 2018;121(11): 1400–8.

104. Friedman M, Jacobowitz O, Hwang MS, et al. Targeted hypoglossal nerve stimulation for the treatment of obstructive sleep apnea: six-month results. Laryngoscope 2016;126:2618–23.

105. Lewis R, Pételle B, Campbell MC, et al. Implantation of the nyxoah bilateral hypoglossal nerve stimulator for obstructive sleep apnea. Laryngoscope Investig Otolaryngol 2019;4(6):703–7.

106. Eastwood PR, Barnes M, MacKay SG, et al. Bilateral hypoglossal nerve stimulation for treatment of adult obstructive sleep apnoea. Eur Respir J 2020; 55(1):1901320.

107. Heiser C, Maurer JT, Hofauer B, et al. Outcomes of upper airway stimulation for obstructive sleep apnea in a multi-center German post-market study. Otolaryngol Head Neck Surg 2017;156(2):378–84.

Obstructive Sleep Apnea and Cardiovascular Disease

Joseph A. Diamond, MD*, Haisam Ismail, MD

KEYWORDS

- Obstructive sleep apnea • Hypertension • Atrial fibrillation
- Premature ventricular contractions • Ventricular tachycardia • Nondipper
- Polysomnography

KEY POINTS

- Obstructive sleep apnea (OSA) is due to repetitive interruptions of ventilation each lasting for more than 10 seconds during sleep as a result of upper airway obstruction and resulting in increased respiratory effort.
- Normally, there is a 10% to 20% decrease in sleep blood pressure (BP) compared with wake BP (dip) on 24-hour ambulatory BP monitoring; however, individuals with OSA typically have an absent dip or paradoxic increase (reverse dip) in sleep period BP.
- The definitive diagnosis of OSA is made by polysomnography, a sleep study that may be performed in a sleep laboratory or at home.
- Clinical trials demonstrate modest reduction of BP with continuous positive airway pressure (CPAP).
- Treatment of OSA with CPAP is necessary for proper management of atrial fibrillation and maintenance sinus rhythm.

INTRODUCTION AND BACKGROUND

Obstructive sleep apnea (OSA) presents as repetitive interruptions of ventilation each lasting for more than 10 seconds during sleep as a result of upper airway obstruction and resulting in increased respiratory effort.[1] This is in contradistinction to central sleep apnea in which there is a loss of ventilatory drive, with a greater than 10-second pause in ventilation, but with no associated increase in respiratory effort. In this article, we explore the relationship between OSA and cardiovascular disease. Observational studies have associated OSA with hypertension often resistant to medication, coronary heart disease, cardiac arrhythmia (particularly atrial fibrillation), and heart failure.

Department of Cardiology, Long Island Jewish Hospital, Northwell Health, 270-05 76th Avenue Room 2008, New Hyde Park, NY 11040, USA
* Corresponding author.
E-mail address: jdiamond@northwell.edu

Clin Geriatr Med 37 (2021) 445–456
https://doi.org/10.1016/j.cger.2021.04.006
0749-0690/21/© 2021 Elsevier Inc. All rights reserved.

PREVALENCE OF OBSTRUCTIVE SLEEP APNEA

OSA is a common worldwide problem. Population-based studies suggest the prevalence of OSA to be 3% to 7% for adult men and 2% to 5% for adult women in the general population, although higher in different population subsets, such as overweight or obese people and older individuals.[2] In a meta-analysis of 17 studies, Benjafield and colleagues[3] estimated that 936 million adult men and women aged 30 to 69 years worldwide have mild to severe OSA, with the highest prevalence exceeding 50% in some locations. Men are 3 times more likely than women to have OSA, and the prevalence increases with age, particularly in those older than 60 years. Patients with OSA are often obese and have an increased prevalence of other cardiovascular risk factors, such as hypertension and type 2 diabetes mellitus. Approximately 50% of patients with OSA have high blood pressure (BP), and up to 30% of hypertensive individuals may have OSA. Although OSA is associated with obesity, significant sleep-disordered breathing is more likely to be the sole cause of elevated BP in relatively lean versus obese individuals. Even minimal degree of sleep-disordered breathing can increase BP and may contribute to hypertension in 5% of hypertensive individuals.[4,5] The association between OSA and hypertension appears to be particularly prominent in patients with resistant hypertension. In one study, OSA was found in 71% of individuals with resistant hypertension, compared with 38% of individuals with controlled systemic hypertension.[6]

PATHOPHYSIOLOGY OF CARDIOVASCULAR DISEASE WITH OBSTRUCTIVE SLEEP APNEA

It is not clear if OSA causes cardiovascular disease or is only associated with cardiac disease, because the 2 conditions share independent risk factors, such as age and obesity. Intermittent hypoxia from OSA causes changes in oxygen concentration, carbon dioxide concentration, and blood pH, resulting in an increase in catecholamine production. Catecholamine production may be further enhanced in response to chronic sleep deprivation. Furthermore, carotid chemoreceptors are stimulated producing a vasomotor center reflex, which with increased catecholamines results in an increase in total peripheral resistance. The cyclic ventilatory pattern of sleep apnea also causes tachycardia and increased venous return, leading to an increase in cardiac output. The combination of increased total peripheral resistance and cardiac output promotes hypertension. The increase in catecholamines and heart rate contributes to tachyarrhythmias and heart failure. In addition to sympathetic excitation, intermittent hypoxia promotes inflammation, oxidative stress, and metabolic dysregulation, all of which promote atherosclerosis, myocardial ischemia, cerebrovascular ischemia, left ventricular hypertrophy, and heart failure.[7]

CLINICAL PRESENTATION OF OBSTRUCTIVE SLEEP APNEA WITH CARDIOVASCULAR DISEASE

Early recognition of the symptoms and signs of OSA is important to initiate treatment before the development of significant cardiovascular disease. Clinical features suggestive of OSA include witnessed gasping during sleep, morning headaches, excessive daytime somnolence, loud snoring, and neck circumference greater than 16 inches (40.6 cm).[8] Screening questionnaires for OSA, such as the Berlin Questionnaire, STOP- Bang Questionnaire, or the Epworth Sleepiness Scale may be helpful, but have varying degrees of accuracy. Features of the physical examination suggestive of OSA include large neck circumference, high body mass index, posterior chin position (retrognathia), reduced distance and increased angles from the chin to the thyroid cartilage, narrow oropharyngeal opening (pharyngeal crowding), macroglossia, chronic nasal or sinus congestion (eg, by trans-illumination), and a deviated nasal septum. Twenty-four–hour ambulatory BP monitoring may be done to assess for changes in the pattern of BP. Normally, there is a 10% to 20% decrease in sleep BP compared with wake BP (dip). Individuals with OSA typically have an absent dip or paradoxic increase (reverse dip) in sleep period BP (**Fig. 1**). The definitive diagnosis is made by polysomnography, a sleep study that may be performed in a sleep laboratory or at home. These studies quantify the amount of apneic events in which there is complete obstruction of airflow for at least 10 seconds, as well as the number of hypopneic episodes, in which there is partial obstruction of airflow with oxygen desaturation of at least 3% lasting for 10 seconds or more. By measuring these events, an apnea-hypopnea index is calculated by adding all apneas and hypopneas and then dividing by total sleep time. An apnea-hypopnea index of 15 or more events per hour, or 5 or more events per hour in the presence of symptoms or cardiovascular comorbidities, is diagnostic for OSA.[7] An example of an apneic event during polysomnography is illustrated in **Fig. 2**.[9]

IMPACT OF TREATMENT OF OBSTRUCTIVE SLEEP APNEA ON CARDIOVASCULAR DISEASE

Lifestyle modifications may be considered the initial treatment for mild OSA. Obesity results in fatty deposits around the neck, which contribute to pharyngeal collapse.

Weight loss may decrease critical closing pressures of the airway and be curative for some individuals, but is very difficult to achieve and maintain. Behavioral therapy

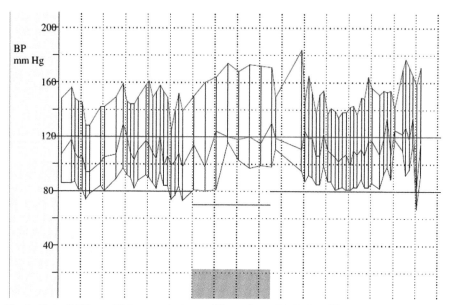

Fig. 1. Plot of BP from 24-hour ambulatory BP monitor with BP in millimeters on the vertical (y-axis) and time on the horizontal (x-axis). The sleep period is represented by a gray rectangle on the x-axis. Each systolic, mean diastolic BP reading is connected by a vertical line. Mean wake period BP is 150/88 ± 12/10 mm Hg. Mean sleep period BP is 166/94 mm Hg ± 9/14 mm Hg. This is a paradoxic BP response or reverse dip.

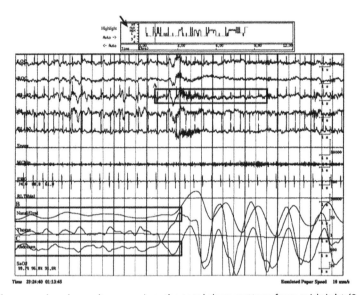

Fig. 2. The upper box (*arrow*) summarizes the total sleep pattern from midnight (0.00 hour) to 9:00 AM (AWK = awake, REM = rapid-eye movement, and sleep stages 1–4). The frequent spikes indicate a disruptive sleep pattern. The vertical line between 0.00 hour and 3:00 AM is detailed in the figure (1:13 AM). It is represented in the first 5 lines by electroencephalogram (EEG) tracings, followed by the nasal/oral airflow tracing, the thorax and abdomen motion tracings, and the oxygen saturation measurements in the lower left corner of the illustration. The nasal/oral airflow tracing shows significant absence of airflow in the boxed region labeled B. There is also paradoxic motion of the abdomen as compared with the motion of the thorax (illustrated in box C). These findings indicate obstructive airflow. Oxygen saturation decreases from 99.7% to 91.8%. Immediately after this period is a sudden increase in airway movement on the nasal/oral tracing with concomitant arousal signals on the EEG tracings (illustrated in the box labeled A). The abdominal and thoracic movement tracings are now synchronized. Over the course of this polysomnography, 68 of these apneic episodes were recorded.

includes avoidance of alcohol before going to sleep, avoidance of sedative use, avoidance of sleep deprivation, and sleeping in a lateral position, thus avoiding the supine position, in which upper airway obstruction occurs most commonly. Mandibular advancement devices hold the mandible slightly down and forward relative to the natural, relaxed position and this results the tongue being farther away from the back of the airway. This may relieve apnea or improve breathing for some individuals. One meta-analysis of 51 studies of patients with hypertension and OSA reported that compared with patients on placebo or not receiving therapy, mandibular advancement devices were associated with a small, but significant reduction in both systolic BP and diastolic BP to levels similar to what is seen with continuous positive airway pressure (CPAP).[10] CPAP remains the first-line treatment for OSA. Randomized trials and meta-analyses have found that effective treatment of OSA using CPAP reduces BP, regardless of whether the patients are hypertensive at baseline. However, the reduction in systemic BP due to positive airway pressure therapy is usually small. In a 2014 meta-analysis that included 30 randomized trials and more than 1900 patients, CPAP therapy was associated with a mean net lowering in systolic BP of 2.6 mm Hg.[11] The 2017 American College of Cardiology/American Heart Association (ACC/AHA) Guidelines indicate in adults with hypertension and OSA, that the effectiveness of

CPAP to reduce BP is not well established.[12] The BP lowering effect of CPAP may be less than that observed with antihypertensive medication. In a randomized crossover trial of 23 patients with both untreated hypertension and untreated OSA, antihypertensive medication (valsartan 160 mg per day) lowered mean 24-hour BP significantly more than CPAP therapy (-9.0 vs -2.1 mm Hg).[13] In another small randomized clinical trial, spironolactone reduced the severity of OSA and reduced BP in individuals with resistant hypertension and with moderate-to-severe OSA. Thirty patients were enrolled in a prospective, randomized, open trial, with 15 in the treatment group, receiving 20 to 40 mg daily of spironolactone in addition to their usual antihypertensive therapy and 15 receiving usual therapy. After 12 weeks of follow-up, apnea-hypopnea index, hypopnea index, oxygen desaturation index, clinical BP, ambulatory BP, and plasma aldosterone level were reduced significantly in the spironolactone-treated group compared with the control group.[14] This study suggested a potential role for spironolactone not only as a treatment for hypertension, but also as a treatment for OSA. Observational data suggest that treatment of OSA with positive airway pressure may reduce the incidence of cardiovascular events, including events related to coronary artery disease; however, this has not yet been confirmed by randomized clinical trials.[15] In one multicenter randomized trial of 725 patients with moderate-to-severe OSA, but no history of cardiovascular events, randomly assigned to receive CPAP therapy or no active intervention, there was no significant difference in the rate of systemic hypertension or cardiovascular events (nonfatal myocardial infarction, nonfatal stroke, transient ischemic attack, hospitalization for unstable angina/arrhythmia, or cardiovascular death) after a median follow-up of 4 years.[16] Surgical approaches to OSA include uvulo-palato-pharyngoplasty (UPPP) and genio-glossal/mandibular advancement in adults, and tonsillectomy/adenoidectomy in children. UPPP is often ineffective, with up to 50% recurrence rate of OSA in 2 years. This procedure should be used only as a last resort except in patients with severe, specific craniofacial abnormalities.[17] Bariatric surgery in obese patients with OSA may result in improvement in more than 75% of patients and a remission rate of 40% after 2 years.[18]

ELECTROPHYSIOLOGICAL EFFECTS OF OBSTRUCTIVE SLEEP APNEA
Atrial Fibrillation and Obstructive Sleep Apnea

Atrial fibrillation (AF) is the most common cardiac arrhythmia in the general population with a prevalence of 1% to 2%.[19,20] The prevalence increases with age to more than 30% of individuals older than 80 years.[21,22] AF carries significant morbidity, mortality, and health care costs. OSA is exceedingly prevalent in patients with AF.[23] Adults with OSA have almost 2 to 4 times increased risk of developing AF.[24] Similarly, adults with AF have a high prevalence of OSA reported in some trials up to 39%.[25–27] As noted previously with respect to hypertension, OSA may not be the cause of AF in all of these individuals. Their coexistence may in part be due to common risk factors, including advanced age, obesity, diabetes, hypertension, and structural heart disease. The relationship between AF and OSA is multifactorial; however, there may a direct causal relationship that is mutually perpetuating. A significant independent association between the 2 disorders exists.[28] This includes sympathetic and parasympathetic system regulation and cardiac electrical and structural remodeling, particularly of the atria, as shown in **Fig. 3**.[29–31]

During an apneic episode, when there is collapse of the pharyngeal airway leading to interruption of ventilation, vagal efferent output is enhanced, which leads to transient bradycardia as well as a shortened atrial effective refractory period. Episodic hypoxemia during sleep apnea in animal models results in surges of the sympathetic

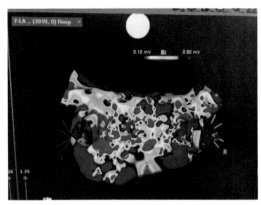

Fig. 3. The posterior wall of the left atrium in a patient with OSA presenting for an AF abla-tion. There are patchy areas of low voltage as shown by the shades of red and yellow compared with the purple areas of normal voltage.

nervous system, thus reducing the induction threshold for AF.[32] However, the patho-physiology is beyond just neurohormonal activation. Sympathetic ganglion blockade provides only incomplete protection against AF associated with apnea.[33–35] There is also electrical and structural remodeling of atrial tissue due to stretch mediated short-ening of atrial refractoriness with resultant susceptibility to excitatory stimuli. Further-more, collagen deposition and changes in gap junction function have been described in individuals with OSA.[36,37] Repetitive apneic episodes resulting in exaggerated changes in intrathoracic pressure lead to left atrial dilatation and fibrosis.[38,39] Electro-physiology studies of these atria in patients with OSA show areas of slow conduction, reduced atrial electrogram amplitude, and complex fractionated atrial electrograms, correlating with the electrical remodeling, as shown in **Fig. 3**. Atrial electrical remod-eling, structural remodeling, and neuro-hormonal activation during apneic episodes provide the milieu for the induction of AF.[36,37] Treatment of AF is more difficult in pa-tients with OSA. In the ORBIT-AF trial, patients with OSA had significantly worse symptoms and were more likely to be on rhythm control therapy.[40] Individuals with OSA had more episodes of recurrent AF, even after catheter ablation.[41–44] Treatment of OSA is indispensable for proper management of AF and maintenance of sinus rhythm. The cohort of patients treated with CPAP in the ORBIT-AF trial were less likely to progress to persistent AF compared with those not treated with CPAP.[11] In addition, other trials have shown less AF after catheter ablation in those patients with OSA treated with CPAP compared with a 57% risk of recurrence of AF in those not treated with CPAP.[43]

Current guidelines recommend treating OSA with CPAP for rhythm control of AF, particularly after catheter ablation. It is especially important in diagnosing and treating suspected OSA in any patient who presents with symptomatic AF and is a candidate for ablation.[45] Suspected OSA should be evaluated in those individuals with drug-refractory AF and those with recurrent AF after cardioversion or catheter ablation.

Premature Ventricular Contractions, Nonsustained Ventricular Tachycardia, and Obstructive Sleep Apnea

Most studies focus on the relationship of AF with OSA. However, there is an increasing body of evidence linking OSA with ventricular arrhythmias (VAs), particularly prema-ture ventricular contractions (PVCs) and nonsustained ventricular tachycardia

(NSVT). VAs have been reported in up to two-thirds of patients with OSA.[46–48] VAs are more common during apneic episodes.[49–51] The mechanisms are similar to those causing the induction of AF in adults with OSA. As with AF, neurohormonal changes, such as enhanced parasympathetic activation during, and sympathetic surges create the arrhythmogenic substrate necessary for VAs.[48] Exaggerated intrathoracic pressure changes cause myocardial stretch, leading to the structural changes in the ventricles similar to the atria. Increased systemic inflammation and endothelial dysfunction from repetitive apneic episodes may directly trigger VAs. These mechanisms also lead to hypertension, ventricular hypertrophy, myocardial fibrosis, ventricular dysfunction, and coronary artery disease, all of which may further predispose these patients to arrhythmia.[52] The frequency of PVCs correlates with the degree of sympathetic tone during waking hours. PVC frequency decreases during normal rapid-eye movement (REM) sleep. Thus, sympatho-vagal balance plays a role in the frequency of PVCs in adults with OSA.[53] NSVT may also be seen with OSA; however, not to the same degree as with PVCs. Abe and colleagues[54] showed that PVCs are more frequent in the more severe forms of OSA. NSVT, however, is not consistently more common in patients with OSA. One study by Mehra and colleagues[55] did find NSVT to be more common in individuals with sleep-disordered breathing (SDB). However, PVCs and OSA have a stronger link. Furthermore, Koshino and colleagues[56] found that 51% of individuals with idiopathic PVCs without heart failure were found to have OSA. This strengthens the idea that of all the VAs, PVCs were more clearly associated with OSA. Other VAs do occur. A study of intracardiac defibrillator (ICD) therapy, including shocks and antitachycardia pacing, in patients with SDB found that VAs were more common during apnea/hypopnea than with normal breathing.[57,58] The presence of SDB was an independent predictor of ICD therapy and the severity of OSA correlated with an increased risk of VAs.[59]

Sudden Cardiac Death and Obstructive Sleep Apnea

In 2005, a study by Gami and colleagues[60] looked at the association of OSA and sudden cardiac death (SCD). The investigators reviewed the death certificates of 112 people who died during sleep and found that 46% of those who died between midnight and 6 AM had OSA. In 2013, a longitudinal study of 10,000 patients found that VAs were not the sole cause of death in patients with OSA. Acute myocardial infarction and pulmonary embolism were also included.[61]

SINUS NODE DYSFUNCTION, ATRIOVENTRICULAR BLOCK, AND OBSTRUCTIVE SLEEP APNEA

Sinus node dysfunction and atrioventricular (AV) block have been linked to patients with OSA. The mechanism is similar to that attributed to AF and VAs, involving electrical and structural remodeling of the myocardial tissue. Fibrosis and dilation of the atria provoke areas of low voltage and slow conduction, resulting in sinus node dysfunction and AV block. Simantirakis and colleagues[62] reported a 22% prevalence of bradycardia with significant pauses on implantable loop recorders in patients with OSA. An observational study by Garrigue and colleagues,[63] showed a 59% prevalence of undiagnosed OSA in patients with permanent pacemakers. Becker and colleagues, found AV block and sinus arrest in 30% of patients with OSA.[64]

There is currently no conclusive evidence that connects the prevalence or severity of electrophysiological effects, including AF, VAs, heart block, and SCD with the treatment of OSA. However, there have been observational trials suggesting that CPAP is an effective strategy in limiting the arrhythmogenic complications of OSA. Larger prospective trials are needed to firmly establish the true role of CPAP in limiting the electrophysiological sequelae of OSA.

CLINICS CARE POINTS

- OSA may be a cause of resistant hypertension.
- OSA is a contributing factor in patients with atrial fibrillation, PVCs and NSVT.
- OSA may be diagnosed with polysomnography.
- OSA may cause a blunted or paradoxical increase in sleep BP.
- Spironolactone may provide benefit for OSA independent of BP lowering effect.
- Treatment of OSA with CPAP may help lower BP, and help maintain sinus rhythm in patients with atrial fibrillation.

DISCLOSURE

The authors have nothing to disclose

REFERENCES

1. Somers VK, White DP, Amin RA, et al. Sleep apnea and cardiovascular disease: an American Heart Association/American College of Cardiology Foundation scientific statement from the American Heart Association council for high BP research professional education committee, council on clinical cardiology, stroke council, and council on cardiovascular nursing. J Am Coll Cardiol 2008;52: 686–717.
2. Punjabi NM. The epidemiology of adult obstructive sleep apnea. Proc Am Thorac Soc 2008;5(2):136–43.
3. Benjafield AV, Ayas NT, Eastwood P, et al. Estimation of the global prevalence and burden of obstructive sleep apnea: literature-based analysis. Lancet Respir Med 2019;7(8):687–98.
4. Young T, Peppard P, Palta M, et al. Population-based study of sleep-disordered breathing as a risk factor for hypertension. Arch Intern Med 1997;157:1746–52.
5. Nieto FJ, Young TB, Lind BK, et al. Association of sleep-disordered breathing, sleep apnea, and hypertension in a large community-based study. Sleep Heart Health Study. JAMA 2000;283:1829–36.
6. Gonçalves SC, Martinez D, Gus M, et al. Obstructive sleep apnea and resistant hypertension: a case-control study. Chest 2007;132(6):1858.
7. Silke R. Mechanisms of cardiovascular disease in obstructive sleep apnea. J Thorac Dis 2018;10(34):S4201–11.
8. Semelka M, Wilson J, Floyd R. Diagnosis and treatment of obstructive sleep apnea in adults. Am Fam Physician 2016;94(5):355–60.
9. Diamond JA, DePalo L. Resistant hypertension in a young man with asthma. Am J Hypertens 2002;15(2):199–200.
10. Bratton DJ, Gaisl T, Wons AM, et al. CPAP vs mandibular advancement devices and BP in patients with obstructive sleep apnea: a systematic review and meta-analysis. JAMA 2015;314(21):2280–93.
11. Fava C, Dorigoni S, Dalle Vedove F, et al. Effect of CPAP on BP in patients with OSA/hypopnea a systematic review and meta-analysis. Chest 2014;145(4):762.
12. Whelton PK, Carey RM, Aronow WS, et al. 2017 Acc/AHA/AAPA/ABC/ACPM/ AGS/APhA/ASH/ASPC/NMA/CNA guideline for the prevention, detection,

evaluation, and management of high BP in adults: a report of the American College of Cardiology/American Heart Association Task Force on Clinical Practice Guidelines. J Am Coll Cardiol 2018;71(19):e127–248.

13. Pépin JL, Tamisier R, Barone-Rochette G, et al. Comparison of continuous positive airway pressure and valsartan in hypertensive patients with sleep apnea. Am J Respir Crit Care Med 2010;182(7):954.

14. Yang L, Zhang H, Cai M, et al. Effect of spironolactone on patients with resistant hypertension and obstructive sleep apnea. Clin Exp Hypertens 2016;38(5): 464–8.

15. Marin JM, Carrizo SJ, Vicente E, et al. Long-term cardiovascular outcomes in men with obstructive sleep apnoea-hypopnoea with or without treatment with continuous positive airway pressure: an observational study. Lancet 2005;365(9464): 1046.

16. Barbé F, Durán-Cantolla J, Sánchez-de-la-Torre M, et al. Effect of continuous positive airway pressure on the incidence of hypertension and cardiovascular events in non-sleepy patients with obstructive sleep apnea: a randomized controlled trial. JAMA 2012;307(20):2161–8.

17. Sundaram S, Bridgman SA, Lim J, et al. Surgery for obstructive sleep apnoea. Cochrane Database Syst Rev 2005;(4):CD001004.

18. Sarkhosh K, Switzer NJ, El-Hadi M, et al. The impact of bariatric surgery on obstructive sleep apnea: a systematic review. Obes Surg 2013;23(3):414–23.

19. Go AS, Hylek EM, Phillips KA, et al. Prevalence of diagnosed atrial fibrillation in adults: national implications for rhythm management and stroke prevention: the Anticoagulation and Risk Factors in Atrial Fibrillation (ATRIA) Study. JAMA 2001;285:2370–5.

20. Tietjens JR, Claman D, Kezirian EJ, et al. Obstructive sleep apnea in cardiovascular disease: a review of the literature and proposed multidisciplinary clinical management strategy. J Am H Assoc 2019;8:e010440.

21. Marulanda-Londono E, Chaturvedi S. The interplay between obstructive sleep apnea and atrial fibrillation. Front Neurol 2017;8:668.

22. January CT, Wann LS, Alpert JS, et al. 2014 AHA/ACC/HRS guideline for the management of patients with atrial fibrillation: executive summary: a report of the American College of Cardiology/American Heart Association Task Force on practice guidelines and the Heart Rhythm Society. Circulation 2014;130(23): 2071–104.

23. Shahar E, Whitney CW, Redline S, et al. Sleep-disordered breathing and cardiovascular disease: cross-sectional results of the Sleep Heart Health Study. Am J Respir Crit Care Med 2001;163:19–25.

24. Somers VK, White DP, Amin R, et al. Sleep apnea and cardiovascular disease: an American Heart Association/American College of Cardiology Foundation scientific statement from the American Heart Association Council for High BP Research Professional Education Committee, Council on Clinical Cardiology, Stroke Council, and Council on Cardiovascular Nursing. In collaboration with the National Heart, Lung, and Blood Institute National Center on Sleep Disorders Research (National Institutes of Health). Circulation 2008;118(10):1080–111.

25. Albuquerque FN, Calvin AD, Sert Kuniyoshi FH, et al. Sleep disordered breathing and excessive daytime sleepiness in patients with atrial fibrillation. Chest 2012; 141:967–73.

26. Bitter T, Langer C, Vogt J, et al. Sleep disordered breathing in patients with atrial fibrillation and normal systolic left ventricular function. Dtsch Arztebl Int 2009;106: 164–70.

27. Gami AS, Pressman G, Caples SM, et al. Association of atrial fibrillation and obstructive sleep apnea. Circulation 2004;110:364–7.

28. Drager LF, Bortolotto LA, Pedrosa RP, et al. Left atrial diameter is independently associated with arterial stiffness in patients with obstructive sleep apnea: potential implications for atrial fibrillation. *Int J Cardiol* 2010;144:257–259.

29. Leung RS. Sleep-disordered breathing: autonomic mechanisms and arrhythmias. Prog Cardiovasc Dis 2009;51:324–38.

30. Force ESCT, Gorenek B, Pelliccia A, et al. European Heart Rhythm Association (EHRA)/European Association of Cardiovascular Prevention and Rehabilitation (EACPR) position paper on how to prevent atrial fibrillation endorsed by the Heart Rhythm Society (HRS) and Asia Pacific Heart Rhythm Society (APHRS). European Journal of Preventive Cardiology 2016;24(1):4–40.

31. De Jong AM, Maass AH, Oberdorf-Maass SU, et al. Mechanisms of atrial structural changes caused by stretch occurring before and during early atrial fibrillation. Cardiovasc Res 2011;89:754–65.

32. May AM, Van Wagoner DR, Mehra R. OSA and cardiac arrhythmogenesis: mechanistic insights. Chest 2017;151:225–41.

33. Ghias M, Scherlag BJ, Lu Z, et al. The role of ganglionated plexi in apnea-related atrial fibrillation. J Am Coll Cardiol 2009;54:2075–83.

34. Linz D, Mahfoud F, Schotten U, et al. Renal sympathetic denervation suppresses postapneic BP rises and atrial fibrillation in a model for sleep apnea. Hypertension 2012;60:172–8.

35. Linz D, Hohl M, Khoshkish S, et al. Low-level but not high-level baroreceptor stimulation inhibits atrial fibrillation in a pig model of sleep apnea. J Cardiovasc Electrophysiol 2016;27:1086–92.

36. Iwasaki YK, Kato T, Xiong F, et al. Atrial fibrillation promotion with long-term repetitive obstructive sleep apnea in a rat model. J Am Coll Cardiol 2014;64:2013–23.

37. Linz D, Schotten U, Neuberger HR, et al. Negative tracheal pressure during obstructive respiratory events promotes atrial fibrillation by vagal activation. Heart Rhythm 2011;8:1436–43.

38. Drager LF, Bortolotto LA, Pedrosa RP, et al. Left atrial diameter is independently associated with arterial stiffness in patients with obstructive sleep apnea: potential implications for atrial fibrillation. Int J Cardiol 2010;144:257–9.

39. Dimitri H, Ng M, Brooks AG, et al. Atrial remodeling in obstructive sleep apnea: implications for atrial fibrillation. Heart Rhythm 2012;9:321–7.

40. Holmqvist F, Guan N, Zhu Z, et al, ORBIT-AF Investigators. Impact of obstructive sleep apnea and continuous positive airway pressure therapy on outcomes in patients with atrial fibrillation—results from the Outcomes Registry for Better Informed Treatment of Atrial Fibrillation (ORBIT-AF). Am Heart J 2015;169:647–54.

41. Kanagala R, Murali NS, Friedman PA, et al. Obstructive sleep apnea and the recurrence of atrial fibrillation. Circulation 2003;107:2589–94.

42. Naruse Y, Tada H, Satoh M, et al. Concomitant obstructive sleep apnea increases the recurrence of atrial fibrillation following radiofrequency catheter ablation of atrial fibrillation: clinical impact of continuous positive airway pressure therapy. Heart Rhythm 2013;10:331–7.

43. Li L, Wang ZW, Li J, et al. Efficacy of catheter ablation of atrial fibrillation in patients with obstructive sleep apnea with and without continuous positive airway pressure treatment: a meta-analysis of observational studies. Europace 2014;16:1309–14.

44. Ng CY, Liu T, Shehata M, et al. Meta-analysis of obstructive sleep apnea as predictor of atrial fibrillation recurrence after catheter ablation. Am J Cardiol 2011; 108:47–51.
45. Calkins H, Hindricks G, Cappato R, et al. 2017 HRS/EHRA/ECAS/APHRS/SOLAECE expert consensus statement on catheter and surgical ablation of atrial fibrillation: executive summary. J Arrhythm 2017;33:369–409.
46. Guilleminault C, Connolly SJ, Winkle RA. Cardiac arrhythmia and conduction disturbances during sleep in 400 patients with sleep apnea syndrome. Am J Cardiol 1983;52:490–4.
47. Hoffstein V, Mateika S. Cardiac arrhythmias, snoring, and sleep apnea. Chest 1994;106:466–71.
48. Marinheiro R, Parreira L, Amador P, et al. Ventricular arrhythmias in patients with obstructive sleep apnea. Curr Cardiol Rev 2019;15(1):64–74.
49. Shepard JW Jr, Garrison MW, Grither DA, et al. Relationship of ventricular ectopy to oxyhemoglobin desaturation in patients with obstructive sleep apnea. Chest 1985;88(3):335–40.
50. Harbison J, O'Reilly P, McNicholas WT. Cardiac rhythm disturbances in the obstructive sleep apnea syndrome: effects of nasal continuous positive airway pressure therapy. Chest 2000;118(3):591–5.
51. Javaheri S. Effects of continuous positive airway pressure on sleep apnea and ventricular irritability in patients with heart failure. Circulation 2000;101:392–7.
52. May AM, VanWagoner DR, Mehra R. Obstructive sleep apnea and cardiac arrhythmogenesis: mechanistic insights. Chest 2017;151(1):225–41.
53. Muller JE, Tofler GH, Verrier RL. Sympathetic activity as the cause of the morning increase in cardiac events. A likely culprit, but the evidence remains circumstantial. Circulation 1995;91(10):2508–9.
54. Abe H, Takahashi M, Yaegashi H, et al. Efficacy of continuous positive airway pressure on arrhythmias in obstructive sleep apnea patients. Heart Vessels 2010;25:63–9.
55. Mehra R, Benjamin EJ, Shahar E, et al. Association of nocturnal arrhythmias with sleep-disordered breathing: the sleep heart health study. Am J Respir Crit Care Med 2006;173:910–6.
56. Koshino Y, Satoh M, Katayose Y, et al. Sleep apnea and ventricular arrhythmias: clinical outcome, electrophysiologic characteristics, and follow-up after catheter ablation. J Cardiol 2010;55(2):211–6.
57. Fichter J, Bauer D, Arampatzis S, et al. Sleep-related breathing disorders are associated with ventricular arrhythmias in patients with an implantable cardioverter-defibrillator. Chest 2002;122(2):558–61.
58. Anselme F, Maounis T, Mantovani G, et al. Severity of sleep apnea syndrome correlates with burden of ventricular tachyarrhythmias in unselected ICD patients [abstract]. Heart Rhythm 2013;10(5):S190.
59. Zeidan-Shwiri T, Aronson D, Atalla K, et al. Circadian pattern of life-threatening ventricular arrhythmia in patients with sleep disordered breathing and implantable cardioverter-defibrillators. Heart Rhythm 2011;8(5):657–62.
60. Gami AS, Howard DE, Olson EJ, et al. Day-night pattern of sudden death in obstructive sleep apnea. N Engl J Med 2005;352(12):1206–14.
61. Gami AS, Olson EJ, Shen WK, et al. Obstructive sleep apnea and the risk of sudden cardiac death: a longitudinal study of 10,701 adults. J Am Coll Cardiol 2013; 62(7):610–6.
62. Simantirakis EN, Schiza SI, Marketou ME, et al. Severe bradyarrhythmias in patients with sleep apnea: the effect of continuous positive airway pressure

treatment: a long-term evaluation using an insertable loop recorder. Eur Heart J 2004;25:1070–6.

63. Garrigue S, Pépin JL, Delaye P, et al. High prevalence of sleep apnea syndrome in patients with long-term pacing: the European Multicenter Polysomnographic Study. Circulation 2007;115:1703–9.

64. Becker H, Brandenburg U, Peter JH, et al. Reversal of sinus arrest and atrioventricular conduction block in patients with sleep apnea during nasal continuous positive airway pressure. Am J Respir Crit Care Med 1995;151:215–8.

Obstructive Sleep Apnea
Cognitive Outcomes

Arpan Patel, MD[a], Derek J. Chong, MD, MSc[b],*

KEYWORDS

- Sleep-disordered breathing • CPAP • Hypoxemia • Beta-amyloid • Dementia
- Cognitive dysfunction • Reversible cognitive symptoms • OSA

KEY POINTS

- Obstructive sleep apnea (OSA) is a modifiable risk factor for cognitive impairment.
- Executive function, verbal memory, and attention are the cognitive domains typically affected in OSA and appear to correlate with severity of hypoxemia.
- Severe OSA appears to contribute to increased beta-amyloid in the brain, and potentially reversible changes on MRI.
- Cognitive dysfunction may impair the adherence of continuous positive airway pressure (CPAP) for treatment of OSA.
- Treatment of severe OSA with CPAP can slow and even reverse OSA-related cognitive decline.

INTRODUCTION

Cognition includes many domains of brain function, such as language, planning, problem solving, processing speed, various memory types, visuospatial function, attention, recognition and regulation of emotions, and learning.[1] Cognitive impairment is defined as loss of cognitive function in one or more cognitive domains and graded as mild cognitive impairment if there is loss of function in one or more cognitive domains but retained ability to perform activities of daily living, whereas dementia is diagnosed when there is loss of cognitive function in 2 or more cognitive domains to the extent it causes social and/or occupational dysfunction.[1] Cognitive impairment is associated with reduced quality of life,[2] increased health care costs,[3] increased risk of motor vehicle collisions,[4] increased risk of falls,[5] and increased mortality.[6] There are an estimated 5.8 million Americans aged 65 and older with Alzheimer's disease as of 2020,

[a] Department of Neurology, Donald and Barbara Zucker School of Medicine, Northwell Health, 300 Community Drive, Manhasset, NY 11030, USA; [b] Department of Neurology, Zucker School of Medicine at Hofstra/Northwell Health, Lenox Hill Hospital, 130 East 77th Street, 8 Black Hall, New York, NY 10075, USA
* Corresponding author.
E-mail address: dchong2@northwell.edu

Clin Geriatr Med 37 (2021) 457–467
https://doi.org/10.1016/j.cger.2021.04.007
0749-0690/21/© 2021 Elsevier Inc. All rights reserved.

but the cohort may grow to 13.8 million in just a few decades.[7] Although cognitive impairment has a high prevalence in the community, it is remarkably underdiagnosed. A recent meta-analysis of 23 studies found 90% of patients in middle-income countries and about 60% of patients in high-income countries have undetected dementia.[8] The standard approach is to search for reversible causes of cognitive impairments, and sleep disturbances should be high on this list.[1,9]

SLEEP DISORDERS AND COGNITION

Sleep deprivation and fragmentation of sleep have been associated with cognitive impairments. High-performing high school students saw significant declines in attention, working memory, and executive functioning with just 1 week of sleep deprivation compared with controls.[10] With the known poorer quality and duration of sleep seen with advancing age, this would be expected to be amplified in the aging brain.[11]

A meta-analysis showed patients with sleep-disordered breathing had worsened executive functioning and were more likely to have cognitive difficulties develop in life.[12] An increase in stage 1 sleep, a sign of sleep fragmentation, significantly worsened scores of attention and psychomotor function.[13] Interestingly, mood appears to be particularly sensitive to sleep deprivation, even more than cognition and motor performance, which is another important mimic of dementia in elderly patients.[14]

OBSTRUCTIVE SLEEP APNEA AND COGNITION: EARLY CONTROVERSY

Obstructive sleep apnea (OSA) causes sleep fragmentation but in addition is associated with gas exchange abnormalities, namely hypoxemia and hypercarbia. Until recently, there was controversy whether the association between OSA and cognitive dysfunction even existed. Strong associations between OSA and development of cognitive dysfunction in some studies[15–17] were countered by others with weak or absence of association.[18,19] The difference was partly explained by differences in assessment tools used and cognitive domains tested.[12,20] Recently published systemic reviews and meta-analyses are reinforcing strong associations between OSA and development of cognitive dysfunction.[12,21,22] One such meta-analysis, which included 14 studies with 4,288,419 patients, concluded that patients with OSA were 26% more likely to develop cognitive dysfunction.[12] Another meta-analysis of 19,946 patients from 6 cohort studies found that OSA is an independent risk factor for developing cognitive dysfunction.[22]

Obstructive Sleep Apnea and Cognition in the General Population

OSA is a relatively common and treatable condition that has been linked as an independent risk factor for morbidity and mortality associated with a wide range of cardiovascular comorbidities, strokes, and metabolic syndrome.[23] Although mental clouding is a commonly known presenting complaint of OSA, and even acute delirium has been reported,[24] less well known are the chronic cognitive impairments related to OSA.

Quan and colleagues[25] found motor and processing speed performance was significantly impaired in a subgroup of OSA patients, which correlated with the amount of time spent hypoxemic below an oxygen saturation of 85%, on home sleep tests. Most importantly, the treatment of OSA may improve and reverse cognitive impairment and dementia symptoms.[26,27]

The double-blinded APPLES study randomized 1098 patients to continuous positive airway pressure (CPAP) versus sham CPAP for 6 months, although patients with neurocognitive complaints or deficits were excluded from evaluation.[27] There was clear improvement not only in subjective measures but also in objective measures of sleepiness. Importantly, there was a signal at 2 months that executive functioning was improved in those with severe OSA treated with CPAP, although this signal compared with controls dissipated at the 6-month timepoint. In a separate analysis of the same population of patients, worse performance in intelligence, attention, and processing speed was associated with the severity of oxygen desaturation.[13] Interestingly, it was not associated with the severity of the apnea-hypopnea index (AHI), but again, patients excluded from the study included those with the most severe cases of OSA, patients with cognitive complaints, those on medications that could affect cognition, and patients with mini-mental state examination (MMSE) scores less than 27. This excluded patient population would have the most to gain and would be easiest to demonstrate improvement with positive airway pressure therapy for OSA. The Sleep Heart Health Study was a much smaller population, and although controlled, was not double-blinded by a sham CPAP arm.[28] However, it did not exclude patients with specific neurocognitive complaints, only those with stroke or organic brain diseases.[28] Similar to others, this study correlated hypoxemia with adverse performance, as motor and processing speeds declined, particularly in those with oxygen saturations dropping to less than 85%.[28]

Cognition, Obstructive Sleep Apnea, and Patients with Neurologic Deficits

Patients with neurologic illnesses may have even higher risks of both OSA and its cognitive impact. In patients with acute stroke, OSA was highly prevalent, nearly 62% to 72%[29,30] in prospectively enrolled patients, and there may be some spontaneous improvements in both cognition and OSA at 1 year poststroke.[29] Even short-term treatment may be useful. In a randomized controlled study of 43 patients after stroke or with transient ischemic attack admitted to a rehabilitation center who were newly diagnosed with OSA (AHI ≥20), the intervention of just 3 weeks of CPAP significant improved attention and calculation compared with untreated controls.[30] In addition, there were trends in improved stroke severity scores, balance, and gait. It has been postulated that OSA could decrease perfusion and oxygenation of the post-stroke penumbra and thus worsen stroke outcomes.[31,32]

In Parkinson disease, OSA prevalence is higher compared with the general population and results in worsening cognitive function if not treated[33]; scores on dementia screening tests improved with sustained CPAP treatment over 12 months.[34] Likewise, in patients with Alzheimer disease (AD), a meta-analysis found a high prevalence of OSA in these patients in comparison to the general population. AD patients who had OSA had earlier onset by a decade and a more rapid decline in cognitive function,[35,36] which raised interest in the scientific community to explore a bidirectional relationship.[37] This finding is of paramount importance, as OSA is already highly prevalent in the community[38] (17% of men and 9% of women are likely to have OSA between 50 and 70 years of age), and incidence increases with age[38] and will likely become even more common because of the aging population[39] along with worsening OSA risk factors, such as obesity.[40] Despite the high current prevalence of OSA, it remains underrecognized and underdiagnosed. Based on the recent estimation, only 5.9 million adults are diagnosed with OSA, whereas 23.5 million remained undiagnosed.[41] This finding is critical because the longer OSA is undiagnosed and untreated, the greater the risk of missing an opportunity to intervene on a reversible cause of cognitive impairment.

Pathogenesis

The link between severe OSA and cognitive impairment is established, but the mechanisms underlying this association are still being investigated. Various theories have been proposed based on studies on animal models,[42,43] which suggest that cognitive dysfunction in OSA can be attributed to multiple factors, as proposed in **Fig. 1**.[44–47] OSA causes repetitive hypoxia and reoxygenation during the night, causing oxidative stress and vascular inflammation.[46,48] OSA can lead to microvascular disease in the brain,[46,47] systemic atherosclerosis,[46,48] and stroke,[49] adversely affecting blood supply for the brain by disruption of its autoregulation.[50] Recent evidence also suggests that vascular inflammation leads to endothelial dysfunction and disruption of the blood-brain barrier, which further results in damage to the neuronal structure.[44] Evidence exists from other systemic diseases, such as chronic obstructive pulmonary disease, where intermittent hypoxemia has a strong association with the development of cognitive dysfunction, as found in cohort and prospective studies.[51,52]

Although patients with OSA have fragmented sleep because of multiple arousals during obstructive and hypopneic events, the frequent nightly periods of hypoxemia may be doing the most damage by contributing to Alzheimer's disease pathology. Animal studies and human cerebrospinal fluid and PET scan studies now show significant associations between sleep disorders and increased A(beta)-amyloid in the brain, a pathologic hallmark seen in Alzheimer's disease due to decreased clearance and increased deposition of A(beta)-amyloid, leading to neuronal loss.[45,53,54] The association between Aß-amyloid and OSA is particularly intriguing. Serum levels of the

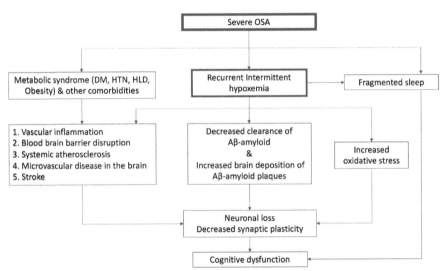

Fig. 1. Proposed mechanisms leading to cognitive dysfunction from severe OSA. Current studies support recurrent hypoxemic episodes as the main factor leading to impaired scores on neuropsychological testing, which may improve with adherence to CPAP. There may be permanent and potentially irreversible changes, as there is preliminary evidence of increased Aß$_2$-amyloid deposition into the brain in patients with severe OSA. OSA is also associated with many comorbidities that also contribute to neurovascular disease, potentially leading to multi-infarct dementia and/or larger strokes, which will increase the burden of neuronal loss and cognitive impairment. Finally, sleep deprivation and fragmentation have been shown to cause cognitive and mood dysfunction even in youth, irrespective of OSA, and likely are another factor in the dysfunction seen in the OSA population, but it is unclear whether they result in structural neuronal changes. DM, diabetes mellitus; HLD, hyperlipidemia; HTN, hypertension.

Aß and P-tau protein, another maker of AD, were found to be significantly elevated in patients with OSA compared with controls who only snored and was positively corelated with the severity of OSA and extent of hypoxemia.[55] This was also recently correlated between severity of OSA (by AHI) and global brain Aß using PET imaging.[54,56]

OSA can also affect sleep-related memory consolidation,[57] which further contributes to cognitive dysfunction. Recent evidence suggests that hippocampal volume loss in patients with OSA[58] interferes with memory and other cognitive functions.[59] Metabolic syndrome (a combination of diabetes, obesity, hypertension, and hyperlipidemia) and other comorbidities can aggravate vascular inflammation and atherosclerosis, which results in microvascular disease in the brain and also increases the risk for lacunar and large strokes,[60] which together results in neuronal loss.

In terms of objective evidence of these impairments, the Canessa group compared 17 newly diagnosed severe OSA patients with 15 age-matched controls using neuropsychology testing and brain MRI voxel-based morphometry, concluding that gray-matter volume losses in the left hippocampus, left posterior parietal cortex, and right superior frontal gyrus improved in conjunction with neuropsychology scores following 3 months of CPAP.[61] These patients were younger (mean 44 years old) without cognitive dysfunction, yet they still significantly improved and then matched controls in memory (list learning, recall, recognition) and tests of attention and executive functioning (improvement in errors), in addition to sleepiness and depression screening. The same research group then reported on white matter signal abnormalities found on brain MRI diffusion tensor imaging that seem specific to severe OSA, discovering that they reversed at the 12-month mark in subjects who adhered to CPAP treatment.[62] The reversal of white matter MRI changes was correlated with normalization of a similar subset of neuropsychological deficits seen in their first study to scores of the control group. Severe OSA should now be considered a reversible cause of cognitive impairments, and in some cases, dementia,[63] and there is evidence for both molecular and imaging data to support pathophysiology and evidence to show recovery.

Cognitive Dysfunction in Obstructive Sleep Apnea: Clinical Relevance

Recent studies have shown that OSA can affect certain components of cognitive function more compared with others. Executive function, attention, verbal/visual long-term memory, visuospatial/constructional ability, and information processing are more likely to be affected, whereas language, psychomotor function, and short-term memory are less likely to be affected.[12,64]

Executive function

Executive function is defined as a set of skills one uses to control and coordinate other cognitive abilities and behaviors.[65] Executive dysfunction was one of the more commonly detected deficits in most cross-sectional and cohort studies.[12,64] Executive dysfunction can be difficult to recognize by patients, their family members, and clinicians. Patients with executive dysfunction have difficulty with starting new or stopping old behaviors, difficulty with planning, organization, prioritization, and inability to multitask.

Patients with chronic medical illness, who are on multiple medications or need physical devices, often have difficulty with self-managing medical care.[66] The medication assessment is crucial for elderly OSA patients, as they may be on multiple medications because of systemic comorbidities and are required to use CPAP regularly Executive dysfunction should be suspected with sudden worsening in OSA symptoms and scores or when patients have difficulty achieving desirable treatment goals despite appropriate attempts and when patients are overwhelmed by disease and treatment regimens.[67]

Verbal memory

Verbal memory is defined as the ability to recall information after it is presented.[68] Recent meta-analysis and systemic review studies[64] showed that immediate and delayed verbal memory were affected significantly in comparison to control groups. The loss of verbal memory will result in difficulty remembering instructions given by medical providers, and if not compensated for, will adversely affect the patient's medical care and patient-physician relationship.[69] If a verbal memory problem is suspected or found, the patient should be given written instructions about their medical care.

Attention

The attention component of the cognitive function of the brain is defined as the ability of an individual to concentrate on a particular stimulus while ignoring other details from the environment.[70] Patients with attention deficits may misplace items, have difficulty with time management, show poor performance in planning and completing a task, and likely lose track of and miss their scheduled appointment.[71] Patients with attentional deficits will have difficulty retaining focus to complete a complex treatment regimen and should be assessed regularly.

In general, patients with cognitive dysfunction may have difficulty with the CPAP ritual. For instance, in a study of patients with Parkinson disease newly started on CPAP, 75% were unable to complete the study because of CPAP intolerance.[72]

Diagnosis

Subtle cognitive dysfunction will often be unnoticed by the patient, family members, and medical providers unless actively sought. The follow-up visits and intake questionnaires should inquire about "mental errors" in addition to losing objects or becoming lost while walking or driving. Routine memory screening, such as the MMSE and Montreal Cognitive Assessment, could be used semiannually to detect early changes of cognitive deficits. Formal neuropsychology testing and neurology evaluation should be requested for patients with suspected cognitive decline. Patients who do not appear to tolerate CPAP may require additional support and attention at the beginning and may specifically require cognitive screening and treatment.

Future Directions

Current guidelines recommend the use of CPAP for moderate to severe OSA, whereas mild OSA has been managed conservatively.[73] However, now that OSA and cognitive dysfunction have an established association, further research should investigate whether patients with mild OSA would benefit from earlier treatment to prevent long-term cognitive decline as well.

Conversely, patients with cognitive complaints and decline should be the focus of future studies of OSA and CPAP, for both short- and long-term outcomes. In the interim, it may be worthwhile to attempt treatment for mild OSA in patients who are exhibiting mild cognitive impairments and dementia.

Based on the current evidence, cognitive impairment in OSA can be considered a multifactorial process, and further research may elucidate the direct mechanism responsible for its pathophysiology to allow for tailored interventions. It is now known that OSA may cause increased amyloid burden on PET imaging, which may be another objective measure to track pathology. Further research should be carried out to find out the utility of brain imaging, including MRI and PET, for the routine surveillance of patients with OSA.

Although OSA may lead to undesirable long-term neurocognitive outcomes, further research can be directed at management of the cognitive impairment, which may adversely affect the care of patients with OSA. Development of a quick screening test to identify the hallmarks of cognitive dysfunction in OSA may be useful for sleep clinics.

SUMMARY

Multiple specific cognitive domains are affected by OSA. Although sleep deprivation is known to cause some cognitive deficits, current evidence highlights hypoxemia as the main culprit in the severity of both cognitive dysfunction and pathophysiology. These studies generally exclude patients with cognitive dysfunction, the patients we are most interested in, so it is possible that milder cases of OSA may also be affected. Studies of patients who already have neurologic disorders, such as stroke, Parkinson disease, and Alzheimer dementia, have identified a high prevalence of OSA that appears underdiagnosed in these populations, and also signals that these patients are even more prone to worsening cognition with progressive OSA, and that treatment may stave off continued decline.

Recognizing cognitive dysfunction is critical in elderly patients with OSA, as it is modifiable and potentially reversible. Appropriate intervention can help with delaying the development of cognitive dysfunction and dementia and sometimes can help in reversing cognitive symptoms if detected early. Simplification of medication regimens and additional support for CPAP utilization may be required to allow successful management of OSA in a patient with cognitive dysfunction, which in itself may be the actual solution to improve the mental status of the patient, and along with it all of the other adverse outcomes of OSA.

CLINICS CARE POINTS

- Geriatricians should be screening patients for cognitive dysfunction in the general population but should additionally consider obstructive sleep apnea as a potential reversible factor in cognitive decline.

- Home sleep tests are simple procedures and widely available. Attended polysomnography may be needed for patients with significant cardiac, pulmonary, or neurologic disease, but the sleep center environment can contribute to disorientation and sundowning.

- Those treating sleep apnea should identify cognitive dysfunction with specific screening questions or tests and refer to neurology or neuropsychology for further testing or treatment.

- The setup, usage, and maintenance of continuous positive airway pressure systems is a complex process that will affect adherence and thus outcome,[74] and patients having difficulty should be cognitively tested and provided more resources to improve adherence.

- With sustained treatment, cognition may improve and along with it the pathologic processes that appear to occur with severe sleep apnea and recurrent hypoxemia.

DISCLOSURE

No conflicts of interest are associated with this publication for all authors.

REFERENCES

1. Arvanitakis Z, Shah RC, Bennett DA. Diagnosis and management of dementia: review. JAMA 2019;322(16):1589–99.
2. Stites SD, Harkins K, Rubright JD, et al. Relationships between cognitive complaints and quality of life in older adults with mild cognitive impairment, mild Alzheimer disease dementia, and normal cognition. Alzheimer Dis Assoc Disord 2018;32(4):276–83.
3. Leibson CL, Long KH, Ransom JE, et al. Direct medical costs and source of cost differences across the spectrum of cognitive decline: a population-based study. Alzheimers Dement 2015;11(8):917–32.
4. Fraade-Blanar LA, Ebel BE, Larson EB, et al. Cognitive decline and older driver crash risk. J Am Geriatr Soc 2018;66(6):1075–81.
5. Tinetti ME, Speechley M, Ginter SF. Risk factors for falls among elderly persons living in the community. N Engl J Med 1988;319(26):1701–7.
6. Bae JB, Han JW, Kwak KP, et al. Impact of mild cognitive impairment on mortality and cause of death in the elderly. J Alzheimers Dis 2018;64(2):607–16.
7. 2020 Alzheimer's disease facts and figures. Alzheimers Dement 2020. https://doi.org/10.1002/alz.12068.
8. Lang L, Clifford A, Wei L, et al. Prevalence and determinants of undetected dementia in the community: a systematic literature review and a meta-analysis. BMJ Open 2017;7(2):e011146.
9. Tripathi M, Vibha D. Reversible dementias. Indian J Psychiatry 2009;51(Suppl 1): S52–5.
10. Lo JC, Ong JL, Leong RL, et al. Cognitive performance, sleepiness, and mood in partially sleep deprived adolescents: the need for sleep study. Sleep 2016;39(3): 687–98.
11. Carskadon MA, Brown ED, Dement WC. Sleep fragmentation in the elderly: relationship to daytime sleep tendency. Neurobiol Aging 1982;3(4):321–7.
12. Leng Y, McEvoy CT, Allen IE, et al. Association of sleep-disordered breathing with cognitive function and risk of cognitive impairment: a systematic review and meta-analysis. JAMA Neurol 2017;74(10):1237–45.
13. Quan SF, Chan CS, Dement WC, et al. The association between obstructive sleep apnea and neurocognitive performance–the Apnea Positive Pressure Long-term Efficacy Study (APPLES). Sleep 2011;34(3):303–314B.
14. Pilcher JJ, Huffcutt AI. Effects of sleep deprivation on performance: a meta-analysis. Sleep 1996;19(4):318–26.
15. Blackwell T, Yaffe K, Laffan A, et al. Associations between sleep-disordered breathing, nocturnal hypoxemia, and subsequent cognitive decline in older community-dwelling men: the Osteoporotic Fractures in Men Sleep Study. J Am Geriatr Soc 2015;63(3):453–61.
16. Ramos AR, Tarraf W, Rundek T, et al. Obstructive sleep apnea and neurocognitive function in a Hispanic/Latino population. Neurology 2015;84(4):391–8.
17. Lutsey PL, Bengtson LG, Punjabi NM, et al. Obstructive sleep apnea and 15-year cognitive decline: the atherosclerosis risk in communities (ARIC) study. Sleep 2016;39(2):309–16.
18. Sforza E, Roche F, Thomas-Anterion C, et al. Cognitive function and sleep related breathing disorders in a healthy elderly population: the SYNAPSE study. Sleep 2010;33(4):515–21.
19. Foley DJ, Masaki K, White L, et al. Sleep-disordered breathing and cognitive impairment in elderly Japanese-American men. Sleep 2003;26(5):596–9.

20. Bucks RS, Olaithe M, Rosenzweig I, et al. Reviewing the relationship between OSA and cognition: where do we go from here? Respirology 2017;22(7):1253–61.
21. Bubu OM, Andrade AG, Umasabor-Bubu OQ, et al. Obstructive sleep apnea, cognition and Alzheimer's disease: a systematic review integrating three decades of multidisciplinary research. Sleep Med Rev 2020;50:101250.
22. Zhu X, Zhao Y. Sleep-disordered breathing and the risk of cognitive decline: a meta-analysis of 19,940 participants. Sleep Breath 2018;22(1):165–73.
23. Bonsignore MR, Baiamonte P, Mazzuca E, et al. Obstructive sleep apnea and comorbidities: a dangerous liaison. Multidiscip Respir Med 2019;14:8.
24. Lombardi C, Rocchi R, Montagna P, et al. Obstructive sleep apnea syndrome: a cause of acute delirium. J Clin Sleep Med 2009;5(6):569–70.
25. Quan SF, Wright R, Baldwin CM, et al. Obstructive sleep apnea-hypopnea and neurocognitive functioning in the Sleep Heart Health Study. Sleep Med 2006;7(6):498–507.
26. Hobzova M, Hubackova L, Vanek J, et al. Cognitive function and depressivity before and after CPAP treatment in obstructive sleep apnea patients. Neuro Endocrinol Lett 2017;38(3):145–53.
27. Kushida CA, Nichols DA, Holmes TH, et al. Effects of continuous positive airway pressure on neurocognitive function in obstructive sleep apnea patients: the Apnea Positive Pressure Long-term Efficacy Study (APPLES). Sleep 2012;35(12):1593–602.
28. Quan SF, Howard BV, Iber C, et al. The Sleep Heart Health Study: design, rationale, and methods. Sleep 1997;20(12):1077–85.
29. Slonkova J, Bar M, Nilius P, et al. Spontaneous improvement in both obstructive sleep apnea and cognitive impairment after stroke. Sleep Med 2017;32:137–42.
30. Kim H, Im S, Park JI, et al. Improvement of cognitive function after continuous positive airway pressure treatment for subacute stroke patients with obstructive sleep apnea: a randomized controlled trial. Brain Sci 2019;9(10).
31. Brill AK, Horvath T, Seiler A, et al. CPAP as treatment of sleep apnea after stroke: a meta-analysis of randomized trials. Neurology 2018;90(14):e1222–30.
32. Duss SB, Seiler A, Schmidt MH, et al. The role of sleep in recovery following ischemic stroke: a review of human and animal data. Neurobiol Sleep Circadian Rhythms 2017;2:94–105.
33. Crosta F, Desideri G, Marini C. Obstructive sleep apnea syndrome in Parkinson's disease and other parkinsonisms. Funct Neurol 2017;32(3):137–41.
34. Kaminska M, Mery VP, Lafontaine AL, et al. Change in cognition and other non-motor symptoms with obstructive sleep apnea treatment in Parkinson disease. J Clin Sleep Med 2018;14(5):819–28.
35. Osorio RS, Gumb T, Pirraglia E, et al. Sleep-disordered breathing advances cognitive decline in the elderly. Neurology 2015;84(19):1964–71.
36. Andrade AG, Bubu OM, Varga AW, et al. The relationship between obstructive sleep apnea and Alzheimer's disease. J Alzheimers Dis 2018;64(s1):S255–70.
37. Piñol G. Impact of obstructive sleep apnea in the evolution of Alzheimer disease. Role of hypoxia and sleep fragmentation. Clinicaltrials.gov, Availble at: https://www.clinicaltrials.gov/ct2/show/NCT02814045. Accessed November 30, 2020.
38. Peppard PE, Young T, Barnet JH, et al. Increased prevalence of sleep-disordered breathing in adults. Am J Epidemiol 2013;177(9):1006–14.
39. Anderson LA, Goodman RA, Holtzman D, et al. Aging in the United States: opportunities and challenges for public health. Am J Public Health 2012;102(3):393–5.

40. Manson JE, Skerrett PJ, Greenland P, et al. The escalating pandemics of obesity and sedentary lifestyle. A call to action for clinicians. Arch Intern Med 2004; 164(3):249–58.

41. Taherian S, Rahai H, Lopez S, et al. Evaluation of human obstructive sleep apnea using computational fluid dynamics. Commun Biol 2019;2:423.

42. Li RC, Row BW, Gozal E, et al. Cyclooxygenase 2 and intermittent hypoxia-induced spatial deficits in the rat. Am J Respir Crit Care Med 2003;168(4): 469–75.

43. Gozal D, Daniel JM, Dohanich GP. Behavioral and anatomical correlates of chronic episodic hypoxia during sleep in the rat. J Neurosci 2001;21(7):2442–50.

44. Lim DC, Pack AI. Obstructive sleep apnea and cognitive impairment: addressing the blood-brain barrier. Sleep Med Rev 2014;18(1):35–48.

45. Spira AP, Chen-Edinboro LP, Wu MN, et al. Impact of sleep on the risk of cognitive decline and dementia. Curr Opin Psychiatry 2014;27(6):478–83.

46. Unnikrishnan D, Jun J, Polotsky V. Inflammation in sleep apnea: an update. Rev Endocr Metab Disord 2015;16(1):25–34.

47. Kepplinger J, Barlinn K, Boehme AK, et al. Association of sleep apnea with clinically silent microvascular brain tissue changes in acute cerebral ischemia. J Neurol 2014;261(2):343–9.

48. Lui MM, Sau-Man M. OSA and atherosclerosis. J Thorac Dis 2012;4(2):164–72.

49. Jehan S, Farag M, Zizi F, et al. Obstructive sleep apnea and stroke. Sleep Med Disord 2018;2(5):120–5.

50. Wang Y, Meng R, Liu G, et al. Intracranial atherosclerotic disease. Neurobiol Dis 2019;124:118–32.

51. Thakur N, Blanc PD, Julian LJ, et al. COPD and cognitive impairment: the role of hypoxemia and oxygen therapy. Int J Chron Obstruct Pulmon Dis 2010;5:263–9.

52. Zhou G, Liu J, Sun F, et al. Association of chronic obstructive pulmonary disease with cognitive decline in very elderly men. Dement Geriatr Cogn Dis Extra 2012;2: 219–28.

53. Kimoff RJ. Sleep fragmentation in obstructive sleep apnea. Sleep 1996;19(9 Suppl):S61–6.

54. Yun CH, Lee HY, Lee SK, et al. Amyloid burden in obstructive sleep apnea. J Alzheimers Dis 2017;59(1):21–9.

55. Bu XL, Liu YH, Wang QH, et al. Serum amyloid-beta levels are increased in patients with obstructive sleep apnea syndrome. Sci Rep 2015;5:13917.

56. Jackson ML, Cavuoto M, Schembri R, et al. Severe obstructive sleep apnea is associated with higher brain amyloid burden: a preliminary PET imaging study. J Alzheimers Dis 2020;78(2):611–7.

57. Kloepfer C, Riemann D, Nofzinger EA, et al. Memory before and after sleep in patients with moderate obstructive sleep apnea. J Clin Sleep Med 2009;5(6):540–8.

58. Macey PM. Damage to the hippocampus in obstructive sleep apnea: a link no longer missing. Sleep 2019;42(1):zsy266.

59. O'Shea A, Cohen RA, Porges EC, et al. Cognitive aging and the hippocampus in older adults. Front Aging Neurosci 2016;8:298.

60. Paoletti R, Bolego C, Poli A, et al. Metabolic syndrome, inflammation and atherosclerosis. Vasc Health Risk Manag 2006;2(2):145–52.

61. Canessa N, Castronovo V, Cappa SF, et al. Obstructive sleep apnea: brain structural changes and neurocognitive function before and after treatment. Am J Respir Crit Care Med 2011;183(10):1419–26.

62. Castronovo V, Scifo P, Castellano A, et al. White matter integrity in obstructive sleep apnea before and after treatment. Sleep 2014;37(9):1465–75.

63. Emamian F, Khazaie H, Tahmasian M, et al. The association between obstructive sleep apnea and Alzheimer's disease: a meta-analysis perspective. Front Aging Neurosci 2016;8:78.

64. Bucks RS, Olaithe M, Eastwood P. Neurocognitive function in obstructive sleep apnoea: a meta-review. Respirology 2013;18(1):61–70.

65. Rabinovici GD, Stephens ML, Possin KL. Executive dysfunction. Continuum (Minneap Minn) 2015;21(3 Behavioral Neurology and Neuropsychiatry):646–59.

66. Feil D, Marmon T, Unützer J. Cognitive impairment, chronic medical illness, and risk of mortality in an elderly cohort. Am J Geriatr Psychiatry 2003;11(5):551–60.

67. Arlt S, Lindner R, Rösler A, et al. Adherence to medication in patients with dementia: predictors and strategies for improvement. Drugs Aging 2008;25(12): 1033–47.

68. Kessels RPC, Overbeek A, Bouman Z. Assessment of verbal and visuospatial working memory in mild cognitive impairment and Alzheimer's dementia. Dement Neuropsychol 2015;9(3):301–5.

69. Hill J. Non-compliance. Lancet 2004;363(9425):2004.

70. Commodari E, Guarnera M. Attention and aging. Aging Clin Exp Res 2008;20(6): 578–84.

71. Torgersen T, Gjervan B, Lensing MB, et al. Optimal management of ADHD in older adults. Neuropsychiatr Dis Treat 2016;12:79–87.

72. Terzaghi M, Spelta L, Minafra B, et al. Treating sleep apnea in Parkinson's disease with C-PAP: feasibility concerns and effects on cognition and alertness. Sleep Med 2017;33:114–8.

73. Littner MR. Mild obstructive sleep apnea syndrome should not be treated. Con J Clin Sleep Med 2007;3(3):263–4.

74. Campbell T, Pengo MF, Steier J. Patients' preference of established and emerging treatment options for obstructive sleep apnoea. J Thorac Dis 2015; 7(5):938–42.

Central Sleep Apnea

Oki Ishikawa, MD*, Margarita Oks, MD

KEYWORDS

- Central sleep apnea • Epidemiology • Diagnosis • Treatment

KEY POINTS

- Central sleep apnea (CSA) is less common than obstructive sleep apnea, but a frequently encountered problem in sleep medicine accounting for about 5% to 10% of clinic patients.
- CSA can be primary (idiopathic), secondary in association with Cheyne-Stokes respiration, drug-induced, or related to medical conditions such as chronic renal failure; or following positive airway pressure (PAP) treatment for OSA (treatment-emergent CSA).
- Male gender, age, heart failure, and chronic opioid use are established risk factors for CSA. Although previously considered as one, stroke is being re-evaluated as a risk factor. High PAP requirement, severe OSA, and mixed central and obstructive events on PSG, are also additional risk factors for treatment-emergent CSA.
- Patients present with symptoms of disrupted sleep or those associated with paroxysmal nocturnal hypoxemia. Consistent history in a patient with risk factors warrants further diagnostic evaluation by polysomnography (PSG). Gold standard for diagnosis is PSG. If home sleep study is suspicious for CSA, PSG should be performed.
- Treatment depends on severity of symptoms but includes optimization of underlying etiology and PAP use. Continuous PAP should be the first PAP modality for CSA. ASV and BPAP ST are second line options available for those with a left ventricular ejection fraction of greater than 45%.

INTRODUCTION

Central sleep apnea (CSA) is characterized by intermittent repetitive cessation and/or decreased breathing without effort. Specific precipitating mechanisms may vary, but it is ultimately rooted in an abnormal ventilatory drive. Although less prevalent than obstructive sleep apnea (OSA), it is a frequently encountered problem in sleep medicine accounting for about 5% to 10% of clinic patients.[1] CSA can be primary (idiopathic) or secondary in association with Cheyne-Stokes respiration (CSR), drug-induced, medical conditions such as chronic renal failure, or high-altitude periodic breathing.[2]

Department of Pulmonary and Critical Care, Donald and Barbara Zucker School of Medicine at Hofstra/Northwell Lenox Hill Hospital, 100 East 77th Street, 4 East, New York, NY 10075, USA
* Corresponding author.
E-mail address: oishikawa@northwell.edu

Clin Geriatr Med 37 (2021) 469–481
https://doi.org/10.1016/j.cger.2021.04.009
0749-0690/21/© 2021 Elsevier Inc. All rights reserved.

geriatric.theclinics.com

An alternative way to categorize CSA is to classify it as hyper- or hypo-ventilation related.

Most CSA patients (including CSR patients) fall into hyperventilation-related, with the exception of CSA related to drug/substance. Hypoventilation-related CSA occurs in disorders in which there is alveolar hypoventilation because of an absent or diminished wakefulness stimulus to breathe, as can be seen in severe opioid toxicity. This may also occur in the context of central nervous system diseases, neuromuscular diseases, and severe abnormalities in pulmonary mechanics such as kyphoscoliosis. However, central apneas tend to be a minor component of their disease. This article discusses the epidemiology, risk factors, diagnosis, and treatment of CSA and its common subtypes.

EPIDEMIOLOGY AND RISK FACTORS

The risk factors for CSA include age, gender, presence of heart failure (HF), prior stroke, opioid use, and other less common medical conditions including neuromuscular disease. Early observational studies suggested that the prevalence of CSA is higher among adults who are older than 65 years (1.1% vs 0.4%).[3,4] However, larger studies that have included both men and women have failed to show this, and it is unclear whether age alone can be considered an independent risk factor.[5] Bixler and colleagues[6] showed that women have an increased incidence of OSA after menopause compared with men, but also showed a paucity of CSA patients among women. It is possible that older individuals are simply more likely to have conditions commonly implicated in developing CSA such as heart failure and stroke. Age itself may not be a true risk factor for CSA.

As mentioned previously, gender seems to play a clearer role as a risk factor for CSA, with a higher incidence in men compared with women. In the previously mentioned study from Bixler with 1000 women and 741 men aged 20 to 100, the prevalence of CSA was 0.4% among men and zero percent among women. Central apneas were detected in 7.8% of men and only 0.3% of women.[6] It has been suggested that this difference results from hormonal effects on the apneic threshold (AT). Administration of testosterone to healthy premenopausal women showed an increase in the AT, whereas administration of leuprolide in healthy males decreased it.[7,8]

HF is perhaps the most well-known associated condition with CSA, more specifically with CSR pattern (**Fig. 1**). CSR is a distinct subgroup of periodic breathing.

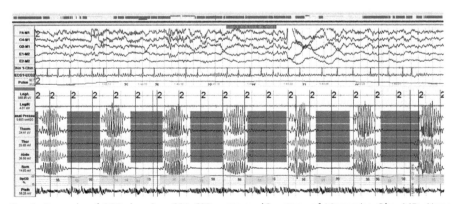

Fig. 1. Example of PSG showing CSA-CSR pattern. (*Courtesy of* Margarita Oks, MD, New York.)

One cross-sectional analysis of a cohort from the Sleep Heart Health study concluded that the overall incidence of CSA in HF patients was 0.9%, with approximately half associated with a CSR pattern.[9] CSR can be observed in both awake and sleep periods, although it is more common in the latter. When it occurs during sleep, it is a form of CSA with prolonged hyperpnea and connotes the presence of a low cardiac output state. The use of the term CSA in patients with HF is synonymous with CSR or CSA-CSR, but it must be noted that it is a distinct subgroup.

The development of CSA-CSR is attributed to the combination of delayed ventilatory response caused by the hypodynamic circulation system, increased chemosensitivity, and reduced end-expiratory lung volume. Initial population-based studies reported that 40% of men with systolic HF had CSA. Subsequent prevalence studies have shown similar percentages, some of which also included women and have shown a similar prevalence.[10,11] Despite overall advances in HF management, this prevalence seems consistent in more recent studies that examined patients with well-controlled HF.[12,13] Although much smaller in sample size, the prevalence also seems to be as high in diastolic failure also.[6]

Risk factors for CSA-CSR in HF patients include male gender, advanced age, atrial fibrillation, and awake hypocapnia.[10] Central events occur most frequently during the lighter stages of nonrapid eye movement (NREM) sleep, particularly after arousals and sleep stage changes. It has been speculated that, because of a generally less stable sleep architecture, male gender is a risk factor for CSA.[10] Interestingly, atrial fibrillation has been shown as a risk factor for CSA but not for OSA despite the well-known association of OSA and atrial fibrillation. Atrial fibrillation can lead to higher left ventricular filling pressures, in addition to the lower ventricular compliance and increased prevalence of pulmonary venous congestion in the elderly population. The additive effects of these cardiovascular changes over time may explain why advanced age is consistently listed as a risk factor for HF patients to develop CSA-CSR.

A form of CSR can also be seen in patients at high altitudes. Altered breathing during non-REM sleep commonly occurs in this situation because of changes in neural signaling caused by hypoxia (caused by a decreased fraction of inhaled oxygen) and alkalosis during sleep from hyperventilation. This phenomenon is called high altitude periodic breathing. This may occur at altitudes as low as 1400 m, but generally does not cause symptoms until above 2500 m.[14] Cognizant of the patient population in discussion, this will not be discussed in depth in this article.

Stroke has been considered as a risk factor for CSA development. Early prospective cohort studies had shown that 70% of patients had developed CSA within the initial 72 hours after the stroke event. However, CSA was detected in only 7% of these patients 3 months later, which may suggest a self-limiting nature of stroke-associated CSA.[15,16] Recent literature has not only supported this self-limiting nature, but also has reported a lower incidence of CSA in stroke patients in general. In a recent meta-analysis of 29 studies that included 2342 patients who had a stroke or transient ischemic attack, sleep-related breathing disorders were identified in 72%, 63%, and 38% of patients when defined as an apnea-hypopnea index (AHI) of greater than 5, greater than 10, and greater than 20 events per hour, respectively.[17,18] Of the studies that distinguished obstructive versus central events, OSA was more common, and only 7% of patients had CSA or Cheyne-Stokes breathing as their predominant abnormality. A recent large cohort-based population study done in the United States also showed a low rate of CSA in stroke patients. Out of the 1346 participants, only 1.4% met criteria for CSA, and the rate of OSA was much higher.

There are other common medical conditions that have been associated with the development of CSA. One of these is chronic kidney disease (CKD). While there is scarce evidence examining CSA and CKD, it is estimated that about 10% of CKD patients have CSA, as opposed to less than 1% for the general public.[19] OSA is also associated with CKD, and evidence suggests that hypervolemia and nocturnal rostral fluid shifts contribute to fluid accumulation in the neck, leading to reduction of upper airway patency and increased collapsibility predisposing to OSA. Also, fluid accumulation in the lungs may stimulate pulmonary chemoreceptors leading to a cycle of hyperventilation and apnea, analogous to the pathogenesis of CSA-CSR in HF patients. This pathogenesis is further illustrated by a small study done by Hanly and colleagues. In this study, Hanly converted 14 patients with end-stage renal disease (ESRD) initially receiving conventional hemodialysis, to nocturnal hemodialysis. There was an overall reduction in the AHI from 46 plus or minus 19 to 9 plus or minus 9 events per hour. The degree of fluid removal and uremia involvement was not elucidated, so it is unclear what extent of effects those had on the reduction of hypopneic events.[20] Subsequent similar studies that examined nocturnal to daytime conversion of peritoneal dialysis and AHI changes after single hemodialysis have shown improvements in obstructive and central events with dialysis. In a study by Lyons and colleagues,[21] the reduction in fluid volume without alteration of uremic status was accompanied by a reduction in chest fluid volume and an increase in transcutaneous $Paco_2$ into the normal range. The removal of fluid potentially reduces respiratory drive and possibly an increase in ventilatory stability via mechanisms explained prior in the context of HF. CKD likely has a role in development of OSA and CSA, and fluid removal likely attenuates the obstructive events.

Another well-known risk factor for development of CSA is chronic opioid use. With the recent increase in opioid use, there is now a growing appreciation for its negative effects including an increased incidence of sleep-disordered breathing (SDB). Opioids decrease central and peripheral responsiveness to hypoxemia and hypercapnia in the awake and sleep state.[22] Although the precise mechanism of CSA associated with chronic opioids is unknown, it may be in part due to the altered ventilatory drive based on this decreased chemoreceptor sensitivity. It must be noted that most studies of opioid related CSA looked at a relatively younger population, with the median age in the third to fifth decade of life. With age-related changes in sleep architecture and higher likelihood of having the associated medical conditions mentioned earlier, the frequency and degree of opioid use affecting sleep may be different.

CSA is the most common sleep-related abnormality diagnosed in chronic opioid users. Although obstructive events may be worsened, there is a larger effect on development of central events in comparison.[23,24] A systematic review by Correa and colleagues[25] revealed that the overall prevalence of SDB ranged from 42% to 85%, with a mean CSA prevalence of 24%. The prevalence of OSA was much higher than that of CSA. This review also identified key risk factors for opioid-induced sleep apnea including a low body mass index (BMI) (16–28 kg/m^2) and a higher opioid dose of morphine equivalent daily dose (MEDD) 200 mg/d or higher. Notably, ataxic breathing was present in 92% patients on MEDD greater than 200 mg/d, and 61% patients with MEDD less than 200 mg/d. Each 100 mg MEDD increased the rate of obstructive apneas by 14.4% and central apneas by 29.2%. Each 100 mg MEDD was expected to increase central apnea index by 2.8 events per hour versus patients not taking opioids. Surprisingly, additive risk with concomitant antidepressant, anxiolytic, and/or ethanol use was not consistently shown.

Use of gabapentinoids (eg, gabapentin or pregabalin) with opioids has been associated with increased odds of opioid related deaths, which in part may be caused by an increased risk of respiratory depression.[26] This was seen more in the elderly population, and one must be cognizant of this potential risk given the frequent use of gabapentinoids in this age group.

Treatment-emergent CSA, previously known as complex sleep apnea, is a distinct entity that surfaces after positive airway pressure treatment (PAP) is begun for OSA. Although reported prevalence is variable, this seems to be detected in approximately 5% to 15% of patients in this scenario.[27,28] Treatment-emergent CSA is defined by the emergence or persistence of central apneic or hypopneic events despite resolution of obstructive events. Whether to treat it as a completely separate entity from OSA is still up for debate based on proposed pathophysiological mechanisms and response to various PAP modes, but it seems to bridge OSA and CSA. This article will focus more on the risk factors, diagnosis, and treatment.

Reported risk factors for treatment-emergent CSA are highly variable, and there are only limited studies that have examined these. Similar to the subtypes discussed previously, male sex, HF, high altitudes, and opioid use have been suggested.[29-31] Potential mechanisms for the development of treatment-emergent CSA include elements such as ventilatory overcompensation to the initial respiratory disturbance of hyperventilation and activation of stretch receptors from PAP therapy. Thus in addition to these risk factors, severe OSA, higher positive pressure, and having mixed obstructive and central events on polysomnography (PSG) have also been identified as possible risk factors.[32-34]

CLINICAL PRESENTATION AND EVALUATION

Elderly patients who have the previously mentioned risk factors with correlating clinical presentation and findings should be evaluated for CSA. Patients will typically present with classic symptoms of disrupted sleep such as excessive daytime sleepiness, poor subjective sleep quality, and difficulty concentrating. They may also report symptoms caused by the repeated nocturnal desaturations including paroxysmal nocturnal dyspnea, morning headaches, and nocturnal angina. Alternatively, CSA may be first suspected when these desaturations are detected in the inpatient setting along with pauses in breathing or arrhythmias.

There are no specific physical examination findings or serologic abnormalities specific for CSA. As such, prudent history taking to evaluate the previously described symptoms is the most reliable screening tool. Because of the insidious onset, these symptoms may go unnoticed, and close evaluation to uncover drowsiness or fatigue during passive monotonous situations (eg, driving, or watching television) is essential. Patients with consistent symptoms and risk factors for CSA should undergo an attended in-laboratory polysomnography (PSG).

Treatment-emergent CSA on the other hand typically is an incidental initial PSG finding during PAP titration for OSA.[35] Central events emerge during the titration, preventing the AHI from normalizing despite decreases in obstructive events. Although less common, treatment-emergent CSA may be detected months after PAP treatment.[27] Although these patients may present with typical sleep-related symptoms, the natural history of treatment-emergent CSA is not well-defined, and how and when to treat these patients remain up for debate.

DIAGNOSIS

As was mentioned in context of the study examining stroke patients, home sleep apnea testing is not yet validated for CSA diagnosis, and PSG remains the gold standard. PSG also helps to elucidate other possible sleep disorders that may be contributing to the patient's symptoms. Various conditions must be considered, including OSA, periodic limb movement disorder, and narcolepsy.

In a standard PSG, various physiologic variables are recorded during sleep and intervening wake periods. Via electroencephalography, electrooculography, and sub-mental electromyography, sleep stages are evaluated. Respiration and effort are measured by muscle activity, airflow, and oxyhemoglobin saturation. Heart rate and rhythm are also measured with continuous electrocardiography. Based on the obtained information, apneic and hypopneic episodes are identified.

Apnea is defined as complete or near-complete cessation of airflow. Scoring an apnea on PSG requires a 90% or greater decrease in airflow (via nasal transducer or oro-nasal thermistor) for a minimum of 10 seconds. A central apnea fulfills this criterion and is associated with the absence of respiratory effort throughout the event. Hypopnea is also a cessation of airflow, but to a lesser degree (decrement from baseline of 30%) and associated with a 3% oxygen desaturation or an electroencephalogram (EEG) arousal. Arousal scoring can have interobserver variability, however; thus a 4% desaturation associated with a 30% decrement in airflow for minimum of 10 seconds is also an accepted definition.[36]

As one can imagine, because of the persistence of thoracic and abdominal movements, distinguishing obstructive and central hypopneas can be difficult. Currently the American Academy of Sleep Medicine (AASM) recommends scoring a hypopnea as obstructive when there are concurrent findings suggestive of upper airway narrowing such as snoring or flattening of inspiratory flow. If these are absent, a hypopnea is scored as a central event.

The remainder of the diagnostic criteria varies based on the type of CSA, and are outlined in **Boxes 1–5**.[2] The absence of hypoventilation is included in some of these. Though hypoventilation can be suggested by hypoxemia on PSG, an objective measurement of CO_2 is needed to ascertain. Hypoventilation is defined by CO_2 levels greater than 55 mmHg or 10 mmHg above the diurnal baseline for at least 10 minutes during sleep. CO_2 levels may be assessed by means of transcutaneous or end tidal monitoring.

TREATMENT

CSA treatment aims to normalize the disordered breathing and prevent sleep-related oxygen desaturations. Whether CSA treatment is indicated at all is controversial. Treatment urgency may depend on the patient's degree of symptoms, with mild cases aiming to treat the underlying associated condition, and severe cases requiring PAP

Box 1
Primary central sleep apnea

PSG reveals ≥5 central apneas and/or central hypopneas per hour of sleep

The number of central apneas and/or central hypopneas is >50% of the total number of apneas and hypopneas

No evidence of CSR

Patient reports sleepiness, awakening with shortness of breath, snoring, witnessed apneas, or insomnia (difficulty initiating or maintaining sleep, frequent awakenings, or nonrestorative sleep)

No evidence of daytime or nocturnal hypoventilation

The disorder is not better explained by another current sleep disorder, medical or neurologic disorder, medication use, or substance use disorder

Box 2
Central sleep apnea—Cheyne-Stokes respiration

PSG reveals ≥5 central apneas and/or central hypopneas per hour of sleep

At least 3 consecutive central apneas and/or central hypopneas separated by crescendo-decrescendo respiration with a cycle length of at least 40 s (ie, CSR pattern)

Number of central apneas and/or central hypopneas is >50% of the total number of apneas and hypopneas

Patient reports sleepiness, awakening with shortness of breath, snoring, witnessed apneas, or insomnia (difficulty initiating or maintaining sleep, frequent awakenings, or nonrestorative sleep)

No evidence of daytime or nocturnal hypoventilation

The disorder is not better explained by another current sleep disorder, medical or neurologic disorder, medication use, or substance use disorder

treatment in addition to that. Optimization of chronic medical conditions such as HF, CKD, opioid use, and central nervous system pathologies may result in the improvement of CSA. Regarding HF, despite medical management advances in its management, optimization has not been shown to resolve sleep-related breathing in this population. Furthermore, outside of cardiac transplant, most studies include HF patients with OSA and CSA, which proposes a challenge in the clinical application of data to those with CSA-CSR only.[37,38] Cardiac transplantation seems to improve but not resolve CSA-CSR, although there have been few recent data.[39,40] Data on left ventricular assist devices are also available, but conflicting in its effect on CSA-CSR.[41–43]

Once a decision has been made to initiate PAP, there are several considerations before choosing the mode. Although there is little evidence on the treatment outcome of individual CSA subtypes, continuous PAP (CPAP) is the preferred initial treatment given the improvement seen in HF patients.[44–47]

Addition of supplemental oxygen is indicated if nocturnal desaturations associated with central events are seen in the PSG. Studies examining CSA caused by HF have demonstrated that supplemental oxygen not only relieves hypoxemia, but may also reduce the AHI.[48] However, these are only shown in relatively small studies

Box 3
Central sleep apnea caused by high-altitude periodic breathing

Recent ascent to a high altitude (typically at least 2500 m, although some individuals may exhibit the disorder at altitudes as low as 1500 m)

The patient reports sleepiness, awakening with shortness of breath, snoring, witnessed apneas, or insomnia (difficulty initiating or maintaining sleep, frequent awakenings, or nonrestorative sleep)

Symptoms are clinically attributable to high-altitude periodic breathing

PSG, if performed, reveals recurrent central apneas or hypopneas primarily during NREM sleep at a frequency of ≥5 per hour.

The disorder is not better explained by another current sleep disorder, medical or neurologic disorder, medication use (eg, narcotics), or substance use disorder

---

Box 4
Central sleep apnea caused by a medication or substance

The patient is taking an opioid or other respiratory depressant

Patient reports sleepiness, awakening with shortness of breath, snoring, witnessed apneas, or insomnia (difficulty initiating or maintaining sleep, frequent awakenings, or nonrestorative sleep)

PSG reveals ≥5 central apneas and/or central hypopneas per hour of sleep; the number of central apneas and/or central hypopneas is >50% of the total number of apneas and hypopneas, and there is no evidence of CSR

The disorder is not better explained by another current sleep disorder

---

(n = 36). A multicenter prospective trial is currently ongoing in the United States, which will further help delineate the appropriateness of supplemental oxygen in these patients.[49] Hypoxemia must be shown to initiate nocturnal supplemental oxygen for patients with awake arterial oxygen tension (Pao_2) of at least 56 mm Hg or arterial pulse oxygen saturation (SpO2) of at least 89%. This will have to fulfill either of the following 2 criteria: (1) a decrease in Pao_2 to 55 mm Hg or below (or SpO2 to 88% or below) for 5 minutes or longer during sleep or (2) a decrease in Pao_2 by 10 mm Hg from baseline (or SpO2 by more than 5% points from baseline) for at least 5 minutes during sleep with associated symptoms or signs attributable to hypoxemia (eg, cognitive impairment, nocturnal restlessness, or insomnia).

If symptoms persist despite CPAP initiation or the patient is intolerant of CPAP, there are other PAP modes that can be utilized. The most important determining factor of which to use is whether the CSA is associated with HF, and what the patient's ejection fraction is. For those whose ejection fraction (EF) is no more than 45%, optimal treatment is uncertain. It is well known and accepted that based on the SERVE-HF trial, adaptive servo-ventilation should not be used for these patients because of the increased all-cause mortality (35 vs 29%; hazard ratio [HR] 1.28, 95% confidence interval [CI] 1.06–1.55) and cardiovascular mortality (30 vs 24%; HR 1.34, 95% CI 1.09–1.65) with ASV use.[50] Supplemental oxygen (if criteria met) combined with optimization of HF may be the optimal approach for these patients.

ASV works by providing a variable amount of positive pressure with a low level of CPAP, with a backup respiratory rate. Bilevel positive pressure with a backup rate (BPAP) works in a similar way by generating a set amount of inspiratory and expiratory pressure with a backup respiratory rate. Although there is no firm contraindication to use BPAP with a backup rate for HF patients with CSA-CSR and EF of no more than 45%, it must be used prudently, given the similar mechanism to ASV. However, for

---

Box 5
Treatment-emergent central sleep apnea

Diagnostic PSG reveals ≥5 predominantly obstructive events per hour of sleep

PSG during the use of PAP (titration or split night study) without a backup rate shows significant resolution of obstructive events and emergence or persistence of central apnea or hypopnea with central hypopnea index ≥5 per hour, and number of central apneas and central hypopneas is ≥50% of the total number of apneas and hypopneas

CSA is not defined by other disorders such as CSA-CSR or opioid related

those whose symptoms are not controlled with medical optimization of HF and nocturnal supplemental oxygenation, this may be the only treatment option.

For patients with an EF of greater than 45% intolerant of CPAP, ASV and BPAP with a backup rate are available treatment options. ASV has been shown to decrease the frequency of central apneas in multiple studies, with a systematic review culminating these results, suggesting a decrease in AHI by a mean of 30 events per hour across 9 trials.[51] It has also been associated with improvements in other parameters such as exercise capacity, EF, and arrhythmic events in patients with implanted cardioverter-defibrillator devices.[52–54] ASV is still considered second-line treatment for CSA, however, because of the EF limitation and lack of direct comparison against CPAP.

Data on BPAP with spontaneous timing (ST) (ie, with backup rate) are scarce and across 2 uncontrolled trials and 1 nonrandomized controlled trial in HF patients with CSA. A meta-analysis of these 3 trials did suggest a mean decrease in the AHI of 44 events per hour, with 1 of the 3 trials reporting an improvement in exercise tolerance.[51] Outside of these 3 trials, data are not available to support or dispute its use for CSA.

Respiratory stimulants such as acetazolamide have been studied in short-term use for treatment of CSA but are not an acceptable treatment option at this time.[55–57] Likewise, several implantable systems have been US Food and Drug Administration (FDA) approved for the treatment of CSA. They involve diaphragmatic pacing to promote normal breathing patterns. Patient selection is of utmost importance if this treatment option is to be pursued.

As mentioned in a previous section, treatment-emergent CSA is a unique entity that is slightly different from the other subtypes of CSA. Most of these patients improve spontaneously after months of CPAP therapy, and may not need any additional intervention aside from optimization of possible underlying etiologies for CSA (eg, HF).[58,59] A repeat PSG or HSAT 2 to 3 months after CPAP initiation should be performed to evaluate for persistence of CSA. If CSA does not improve, either ASV or BPAP ST can be used (provided EF >45%). If these modalities are unavailable because of socioeconomic or logistical issues, then CPAP can be continued to treat the OSA component.

SUMMARY

CSA encompasses a wide range of unstable breathing associated with a wide range of risk factors including gender, HF, and opioid use. It can lead to substantial comorbidity and increased risk of adverse cardiovascular outcomes. Symptom onset is insidious, and prudent history taking, led by high clinical suspicion is paramount to establishing a diagnosis. The underlying pathophysiology and the prevalence of the various forms of CSA greatly vary based on the associated conditions and etiology as demonstrated previously. Treatment approaches should be dynamic, including treatment of these conditions and utilizing various NIV modes depending on the patient population. Studies discussed in this article have highlighted some of the key risk factors, diagnostic approach, and treatment of CSA, but there is still a paucity of data, especially in the elderly population, and further investigation needs to be pursued.

CLINICS CARE POINTS

- CSA is less common than OSA, but a frequently encountered problem in sleep medicine accounting for about 5% to 10% of clinic patients.

- CSA can be primary (idiopathic), secondary in association with CSR, drug-induced, or medical conditions such as chronic renal failure; or following PAP treatment for OSA (treatment-emergent CSA).
- Male gender, age in males, HF, and chronic opioid use are established risk factors for CSA. Although previously considered one, stroke is being re-evaluated as a risk factor. High PAP requirement, severe OSA, and mixed central and obstructive events on PSG are also risk factors for treatment-emergent CSA.
- Patients present with symptoms of disrupted sleep or those associated with paroxysmal nocturnal hypoxemia. Consistent history in a patient with risk factors warrants further diagnostic evaluation by PSG. Gold standard for diagnosis is PSG. If home sleep study is suspicious for CSA, PSG should be performed.
- Treatment depends on severity of symptoms but includes optimization of underlying etiology and PAP use.
- CPAP should be the first-line PAP modality for CSA. ASV and BPAP ST are second-line options available for those with a left ventricular ejection fraction of greater than 45%.

DISCLOSURE

The authors have nothing to disclose.

REFERENCES

1. Muza RT. Central sleep apnoea-a clinical review. J Thorac Dis 2015;7(5):930–7.
2. Sateia MJ. International classification of sleep disorders-third edition: highlights and modifications. Chest 2014;146(5):1387–94.
3. Bixler EO, Vgontzas AN, Ten Have T, et al. Effects of age on sleep apnea in men: I. Prevalence and severity. Am J Respir Crit Care Med 1998;157(1):144–8.
4. Mehra R, Stone KL, Blackwell T, et al. Prevalence and correlates of sleep-disordered breathing in older men: osteoporotic fractures in men sleep study: sleep apnea IN older men. J Am Geriatr Soc 2007;55(9):1356–64.
5. Young T. Predictors of sleep-disordered breathing in community-dwelling adults. The sleep heart health study. Arch Intern Med 2002;162(8):893.
6. Bixler EO, Vgontzas AN, Lin HM, et al. Prevalence of sleep-disordered breathing in women: effects of gender. Am J Respir Crit Care Med 2001;163(3 Pt 1):608–13.
7. Zhou XS, Rowley JA, Demirovic F, et al. Effect of testosterone on the apneic threshold in women during NREM sleep. J Appl Physiol (1985) 2003;94(1):101–7.
8. Rowley JA, Zhou XS, Diamond MP, et al. The determinants of the apnea threshold during NREM sleep in normal subjects. Sleep 2006;29(1):95–103.
9. Donovan LM, Kapur VK. Prevalence and characteristics of central compared to obstructive sleep apnea: analyses from the sleep heart health study cohort. Sleep 2016;39(7):1353–9.
10. Sin DD, Fitzgerald F, Parker JD, et al. Risk factors for central and obstructive sleep apnea in 450 men and women with congestive heart failure. Am J Respir Crit Care Med 1999;160(4):1101–6.
11. Oldenburg O, Lamp B, Faber L, et al. Sleep-disordered breathing in patients with symptomatic heart failure. A contemporary study of prevalence in and characteristics of 700 patients. Eur J Heart Fail 2007;9(3):251–7.
12. MacDonald M, Fang J, Pittman SD, et al. The current prevalence of sleep disordered breathing in congestive heart failure patients treated with beta-blockers. J Clin Sleep Med 2008;4(1):38–42.

13. Tremel F, Pépin J-L, Veale D, et al. High prevalence and persistence of sleep apnoea in patients referred for acute left ventricular failure and medically treated over 2 months. Eur Heart J 1999;20(16):1201–9.

14. Küpper T, Schöffl V, Netzer N. Cheyne Stokes breathing at high altitude: a helpful response or a troublemaker? Sleep Breath Schlaf Atm 2008;12(2):123–7.

15. Bassetti C, Aldrich MS. Sleep apnea in acute cerebrovascular diseases: final report on 128 patients. Sleep 1999;22(2):217–23.

16. Bassetti C, Aldrich MS, Chervin RD, et al. Sleep apnea in patients with transient ischemic attack and stroke: a prospective study of 59 patients. Neurology 1996; 47(5):1167–73.

17. Seiler A, Camilo M, Korostovtseva L, et al. Prevalence of sleep-disordered breathing after stroke and TIA: a meta-analysis. Neurology 2019;92(7):e648–54.

18. Schütz SG, Lisabeth LD, Hsu C-W, et al. Central sleep apnea is uncommon after stroke. Sleep Med 2020. https://doi.org/10.1016/j.sleep.2020.08.025.

19. Lin C-H, Lurie RC, Lyons OD. Sleep apnea and chronic kidney disease. Chest 2020;157(3):673–85.

20. Hanly PJ, Pierratos A. Improvement of sleep apnea in patients with chronic renal failure who undergo nocturnal hemodialysis. N Engl J Med 2001;344(2):102–7.

21. Lyons OD, Chan CT, Yadollahi A, et al. Effect of ultrafiltration on sleep apnea and sleep structure in patients with end-stage renal disease. Am J Respir Crit Care Med 2015;191(11):1287–94.

22. Pattinson KTS. Opioids and the control of respiration. Br J Anaesth 2008;100(6): 747–58.

23. Farney RJ, McDonald AM, Boyle KM, et al. Sleep disordered breathing in patients receiving therapy with buprenorphine/naloxone. Eur Respir J 2013;42(2): 394–403.

24. Wang D, Teichtahl H, Drummer O, et al. Central sleep apnea in stable methadone maintenance treatment patients. Chest 2005;128(3):1348–56.

25. Correa D, Farney RJ, Chung F, et al. Chronic opioid use and central sleep apnea: a review of the prevalence, mechanisms, and perioperative considerations. Anesth Analg 2015;120(6):1273–85.

26. Gomes T, Juurlink DN, Antoniou T, et al. Gabapentin, opioids, and the risk of opioid-related death: a population-based nested case-control study. PLoS Med 2017;14(10):e1002396.

27. Cassel W, Canisius S, Becker HF, et al. A prospective polysomnographic study on the evolution of complex sleep apnoea. Eur Respir J 2011;38(2):329–37.

28. Nigam G, Riaz M, Chang ET, et al. Natural history of treatment-emergent central sleep apnea on positive airway pressure: a systematic review. Ann Thorac Med 2018;13(2):86–91.

29. Lehman S, Antic NA, Thompson C, et al. Central sleep apnea on commencement of continuous positive airway pressure in patients with a primary diagnosis of obstructive sleep apnea-hypopnea. J Clin Sleep Med 2007;3(5):462–6.

30. Morgenthaler TI, Kagramanov V, Hanak V, et al. Complex sleep apnea syndrome: is it a unique clinical syndrome? Sleep 2006;29(9):1203–9.

31. Bitter T, Westerheide N, Hossain MS, et al. Complex sleep apnoea in congestive heart failure. Thorax 2011;66(5):402–7.

32. Younes M, Ostrowski M, Thompson W, et al. Chemical control stability in patients with obstructive sleep apnea. Am J Respir Crit Care Med 2001;163(5):1181–90.

33. Buckle P, Millar T, Kryger M. The effect of short-term nasal CPAP on Cheyne-Stokes respiration in congestive heart failure. Chest 1992;102(1):31–5.

34. Johnson KG, Johnson DC. Bilevel positive airway pressure worsens central apneas during sleep. Chest 2005;128(4):2141–50.

35. Thomas RJ, Terzano MG, Parrino L, et al. Obstructive sleep-disordered breathing with a dominant cyclic alternating pattern–a recognizable polysomnographic variant with practical clinical implications. Sleep 2004;27(2):229–34.

36. Berry RB, Quan SF, Abreu AR, et al, for the American Academy of Sleep Medicine. The AASM Manual for the scoring of sleep and associated events: rules, terminology and technical specifications, Version 2.6. Availble at: www.aasmnet.org.

37. Walsh JT, Andrews R, Starling R, et al. Effects of captopril and oxygen on sleep apnoea in patients with mild to moderate congestive cardiac failure. Br Heart J 1995;73(3):237–41.

38. Dark DS, Pingleton SK, Kerby GR, et al. Breathing pattern abnormalities and arterial oxygen desaturation during sleep in the congestive heart failure syndrome. Chest 1987;91(6):833–6.

39. Mansfield DR, Solin P, Roebuck T, et al. The effect of successful heart transplant treatment of heart failure on central sleep apnea. Chest 2003;124(5):1675–81.

40. Murdock DK, Lawless CE, Loeb HS, et al. The effect of heart transplantation on Cheyne-Stokes respiration associated with congestive heart failure. J Heart Transpl 1986;5(4):336–7.

41. Padeletti M, Henriquez A, Mancini DM, et al. Persistence of Cheyne-Stokes breathing after left ventricular assist device implantation in patients with acutely decompensated end-stage heart failure. J Heart Lung Transpl 2007;26(7):742–4.

42. Harun N-S, Leet A, Naughton MT. Improvement in sleep-disordered breathing after insertion of left ventricular assist device. Ann Am Thorac Soc 2013;10(3):272–3.

43. Vazir A, Hastings PC, Morrell MJ, et al. Resolution of central sleep apnoea following implantation of a left ventricular assist device. Int J Cardiol 2010;138(3):317–9.

44. Naughton MT, Benard DC, Rutherford R, et al. Effect of continuous positive airway pressure on central sleep apnea and nocturnal PCO_2 in heart failure. Am J Respir Crit Care Med 1994;150(6 Pt 1):1598–604.

45. Bradley TD, Logan AG, Kimoff RJ, et al. Continuous positive airway pressure for central sleep apnea and heart failure. N Engl J Med 2005;353(19):2025–33.

46. Naughton MT, Liu PP, Bernard DC, et al. Treatment of congestive heart failure and Cheyne-Stokes respiration during sleep by continuous positive airway pressure. Am J Respir Crit Care Med 1995;151(1):92–7.

47. Granton JT, Naughton MT, Benard DC, et al. CPAP improves inspiratory muscle strength in patients with heart failure and central sleep apnea. Am J Respir Crit Care Med 1996;153(1):277–82.

48. Bordier P, Lataste A, Hofmann P, et al. Nocturnal oxygen therapy in patients with chronic heart failure and sleep apnea: a systematic review. Sleep Med 2016;17:149–57.

49. Javaheri S, Brown LK, Khayat RN. Update on apneas of heart failure with reduced ejection fraction: Emphasis on the physiology of treatment: Part 2: central sleep apnea. Chest 2020;157(6):1637–46.

50. Cowie MR, Woehrle H, Wegscheider K, et al. Adaptive servo-ventilation for central sleep apnea in systolic heart failure. N Engl J Med 2015;373(12):1095–105.

51. Aurora RN, Chowdhuri S, Ramar K, et al. The treatment of central sleep apnea syndromes in adults: practice parameters with an evidence-based literature review and meta-analyses. Sleep 2012;35(1):17–40.

52. Pepperell JCT, Maskell NA, Jones DR, et al. A randomized controlled trial of adaptive ventilation for Cheyne-Stokes breathing in heart failure. Am J Respir Crit Care Med 2003;168(9):1109–14.
53. Oldenburg O, Bitter T, Lehmann R, et al. Adaptive servoventilation improves cardiac function and respiratory stability. Clin Res Cardiol 2011;100(2):107–15.
54. Sharma BK, Bakker JP, McSharry DG, et al. Adaptive servoventilation for treatment of sleep-disordered breathing in heart failure: a systematic review and meta-analysis. Chest 2012;142(5):1211–21.
55. DeBacker WA, Verbraecken J, Willemen M, et al. Central apnea index decreases after prolonged treatment with acetazolamide. Am J Respir Crit Care Med 1995; 151(1):87–91.
56. Javaheri S. Acetazolamide improves central sleep apnea in heart failure: a double-blind, prospective study. Am J Respir Crit Care Med 2006;173(2):234–7.
57. White DP, Zwillich CW, Pickett CK, et al. Central sleep apnea. Improvement with acetazolamide therapy. Arch Intern Med 1982;142(10):1816–9.
58. Javaheri S, Smith J, Chung E. The prevalence and natural history of complex sleep apnea. J Clin Sleep Med 2009;5(3):205–11.
59. Morgenthaler TI, Kuzniar TJ, Wolfe LF, et al. The complex sleep apnea resolution study: a prospective randomized controlled trial of continuous positive airway pressure versus adaptive servoventilation therapy. Sleep 2014;37(5):927–34.

Rapid Eye Movement Behavior Disorder and Other Parasomnias

Maksim Korotun, DO*, Luis Quintero, DO, MPH, Stella S. Hahn, MD

KEYWORDS

- Parasomnias • Elderly • Alpha-synuclein • Neurodegeneration
- Rapid eye movement sleep behavior disorder • Dream enactment behavior
- Rapid eye movement without atonia

KEY POINTS

- Rapid eye movement (REM) behavior disorder (RBD) is a REM parasomnia that occurs primarily in the elderly.
- RBD can be the initial symptom of a neurodegenerative disorder that may only be evident decades later.
- The pathophysiology of the disorder is loss of skeletal muscle atonia in REM sleep and subsequent dream enactment.
- Definitive diagnosis is achieved with a history of dream enactment and an in-laboratory polysomnography showing REM sleep without atonia.
- Treatment of the disorder includes providing a safe sleeping environment and pharmacotherapy (eg, melatonin or clonazepam).

INTRODUCTION

Parasomnias are undesirable physical events or experiences that occur during entry into sleep, within sleep, or during arousal from sleep and can occur during non-rapid eye movement sleep (NREM), rapid eye movement sleep (REM), or during transition to and from sleep.[1]

NREM parasomnias typically occur during N3 sleep, also known as slow wave sleep (SWS). SWS occurs with greater frequency during the first third of the night. Therefore, NREM parasomnias tend to occur earlier in the night. As SWS is the deepest stage of sleep with the greatest arousal threshold, NREM parasomnias are not usually recalled by the patient, who may be difficult to awaken. SWS is maximal in children in whom it can be up to 40% of the night, but a reduction in the amount of this deeper stage of

Division of Pulmonary, Critical Care and Sleep Medicine, Department of Medicine, Donald and Barbara Zucker School of Medicine-Northwell, 410 Lakeville Road, Suite 107, New Hyde Park, NY 11042, USA
* Corresponding author.
E-mail address: mkorotun@northwell.edu

Clin Geriatr Med 37 (2021) 483–490
https://doi.org/10.1016/j.cger.2021.04.008
0749-0690/21/© 2021 Elsevier Inc. All rights reserved.
geriatric.theclinics.com

sleep is seen during adolescence, with a marked decrease seen starting middle age.[2,3] There are reports of complete absence of SWS after 90 years of age.[4] Consequently, NREM parasomnias occur less frequently in older adults.

NREM sleep and REM sleep alternate cyclically throughout the night. The first REM sleep period is short, typically under 10 minutes, but periods become longer as the night progresses, and are longest in the last third of the night. Accordingly, REM parasomnias tend to occur later in the night,[3] in contrast to NREM parasomnias, which are more likely to occur early in the sleep period. Normal REM sleep is characterized by suppression of muscle tone, known as atonia, which is evident on the electromyogram during polysomnography. Most vivid dreaming occurs during REM sleep. The percentage of REM sleep, unlike SWS, is preserved into adulthood.

RAPID EYE MOVEMENT SLEEP BEHAVIOR DISORDER

REM sleep behavior disorder (RBD) is a REM-related parasomnia seen typically in the older population and is characterized by abnormal behaviors emerging during REM sleep because of loss of muscle atonia that is seen during normal REM sleep. This loss of muscle atonia allows for enactment of dreams, which are usually violent and action-filled, and can lead to sleep-related injury of patients or bed partners.[1,5]

Clinical Symptoms

RBD consists of episodes related to dream enactment behavior during REM sleep. These dream enactments may range from vocalization to possible complex motor behaviors.[6,7] RBD occurs in greater frequency in the last half of the night given the increased duration of REM sleep during this time.[3] Enactments may be short in duration but can progress to several minutes. Unlike non-REM parasomnias, patients with RBD are usually able to describe the dream content and recall their enactment behaviors. The dreams are often categorized as fight or flight in origin which may prompt aggressive and repetitive movements (ie, thrashing, punching, kicking, and yelling). Patients may inadvertently harm their bed partners or themselves during this behavior, and may fall out of bed. Individuals diagnosed with REM behavior disorder associated with a degenerative neurologic disorder will exhibit an increase in dream-enactment as the neurologic condition progresses.[6,7]

Epidemiology

The prevalence of RBD varies in the literature. Most population-based studies of REM behavior disorder in the general population show a prevalence of 0.5% to 1.0%.[8] However, in a recent community-based Korean study looking at subjects over the age of 60 years, the prevalence was 2.0%.[9] These numbers may not be reflective of the overall disease burden in the population, as many of the cases are undiagnosed.

Demographic analysis shows a 2-fold increase in frequency in men compared with women over the age of 50. The mean age of diagnosis was 53.7 years old. In addition, men were more likely to exhibit aggressive and violent behavior that would awaken them from sleep.[10]

Diagnosis

To achieve a definitive diagnosis of RBD, the patient should clinically present with symptoms of dream enactment with overnight in-laboratory polysomnography showing evidence of REM sleep without atonia (RSWA). These findings need to be present in the absence of epileptiform activity and with no alternative explanation for the parasomnia (**Box 1**).

Box 1
Diagnostic criteria for rapid eye movement sleep behavior disorder

All of the following must be met:
- Repeated episodes of sleep-related vocalization and/or complex behaviors
- These behaviors are documented by polysomnography to occur during REM sleep, or, based on clinical history of dream enactment, are presumed to occur during REM sleep
- Polysomnographic recording demonstrates REM sleep without atonia[a]
- The disturbance is not better explained by another sleep disorder, mental health disorder, medication, or substance use

[a]On occasion, there may be patients with a typical clinical history of RBD with dream-enacting behaviors, who also exhibit typical RBD behaviors observed on video polysomnography (vPSG), but do not demonstrate sufficient RSWA to satisfy PSG criteria for diagnosing RBD. RBD may be provisionally diagnosed on these patients, based on clinical judgment. The same rule applies when vPSG is not readily available.

Data from Medicine AAoS. International Classification of Sleep Disorders. 3rd edition, 2014.

The gold standard for diagnosis of RBD is to perform an in-laboratory PSG. In addition to the standard monitoring of the chin and anterior tibialis muscle activity, monitoring of the flexor digitorum brevis and biceps brachii can improve the diagnostic accuracy of RSWA in patients who may predominantly exhibit upper extremity behavior during REM sleep. Video recording may obviously correlate motor activity with REM. To diagnose RSWA during REM sleep, more than half of the epoch should exhibit an increase in muscle tone.[11]

In cases where an in-laboratory polysomnography evaluation is not feasible, a concept that is becoming more accepted in clinical practice is probable RBD, which can be diagnosed by using a validated screening tool. The Mayo Sleep Questionnaire includes questions about dream enactment behavior (DEB) for both patient and bed partner and is highly specific for RBD.[12] It is available free to the public and can be downloaded from the Web site: http://www.mayoclinic.org/pdfs/MSQ-copyrightfinal.pdf.[13] In addition, the RBD questionnaire (RBDQ-HK) is a 13-item self-reported screening tool with a moderate sensitivity (82.2%) and specificity (86.9%) for RBD.[14] These questionnaires, although not the gold standard, can be useful in identifying and monitoring patients with reported sleep disturbances and suspicion for RBD. The violent nature of DEB can cause significant injury to patient and bed partner; if a classic history is obtained, empiric treatment may be indicated prior to definitive diagnosis by polysomnography, particularly if this is likely to be delayed.

Normal Rapid Eye Movement Sleep and Pathophysiology

RBD is characterized by loss of skeletal muscle atonia during REM sleep with subsequent dream enactment. During normal REM sleep, there are 2 motor systems involved in stabilizing REM sleep; one is generating REM with atonia or REM-on region and the other being the locomotor generator region responsible for locomotor activity suppression. The REM-on region is comprised of the precoeruleus and sublateraldorsal nuclei (SLD) that work through direct and indirect mechanisms. The direct mechanism has neurons projecting to the spinal interneuron (inhibitory) that acts on the spinal motor neuron to inhibit skeletal muscle activity. The indirect pathway has projections to the magnocellular reticular formation (MCRF), which acts directly on the skeletal muscle to induce inhibition. The locomotor pathway is poorly understood but is thought to project to the spinal motor neuron in an inhibitory fashion.[15]

The proposed pathophysiology of RBD disorder is thought to be neurodegeneration or the deposition of alpha-synuclein at the SLD nucleus, which compromises the direct and indirect pathway pathways of the REM-on region responsible for skeletal muscle inhibition.

Clinical Vignette

62-year-old woman with a past medical history (PMH) of Parkinson disease being treated with carbidopa-levodopa presented for evaluation of excessive daytime somnolence and dream enactment behavior. She noted snoring and had an ESS (Epworth sleepiness scale) score of 15 out of 24 on the initial visit. About 1 year ago, she was noted to be acting out her dreams with her arms flailing and talking in her sleep. On several occasions, she punched and kicked her bed partner while dreaming she was being attacked. She woke up remembering her dream and felt mortified about hurting her husband. These features would occur several times a month and were disturbing to both the patient and her bed partner. Dreams enacted were action-related dreams and she did not fall out of bed or hurt herself during these episodes.

Given the clinical presentation, the patient was referred to the sleep laboratory for an in-laboratory PSG to screen for obstructive sleep apnea (OSA) and evaluate for REM behavior disorder. No clinically significant OSA was evident on the PSG. However, there was evidence of REM sleep without atonia (**Fig. 1**). **Fig. 1**B shows a normal epoch of REM sleep with expected atonia seen.

She was counseled on ensuring a safe bedroom environment and started on melatonin at 6 mg nightly, with good response.

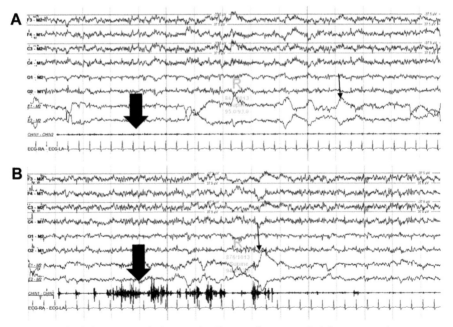

Fig. 1. Standard electroencephalogram (EEG) recording on an in-laboratory polysomnography. (*A*) REM sleep with atonia; black thin arrow: conjugate eye movement; thick back arrow: lack of muscle tone on the chin EMG. (*B*) REM sleep without atonia; black thin arrow: conjugate eye movement; thick back arrow: evidence of muscle tone on the chin EMG.

Treatment

Treatment for RBD is approached in 3 ways: ensuring safety in the bedroom, assessing for reversible causes, and pharmacologic treatment to suppress dream enactment. A survey of patients who had RBD found that 55% of those surveyed reported injury to self or to their bed partners. Providers should suggest making the bedroom a safe environment, which includes but is not limited to: bedrails, lowering the bed, removing night stands, or even having a bed partner sleep in another bed.[6]

Several medication classes are known to elicit iatrogenic RBD and should be reviewed. The classes of medications that are known to cause REM without atonia are selective serotonin reuptake inhibitors (SSRIs), serotonin norepinephrine reuptake inhibitors (SNRIs), tricyclic antidepressants (TCAs), and monoamine oxidase inhibitors (MAOIs). Discontinuation of these medications may lead to the resolution of iatrogenic RBD.

Severe OSA has been shown to destabilize sleep, which can cause dysregulation of the muscle suppression pathways during REM. This can mimic dream enactment and present like RBD (pseudo-RBD). The use of continuous positive airway pressure (CPAP) in patients with OSA can eliminate dream enactment by stabilizing REM sleep.[16] All patients being evaluated for RBD should be treated for OSA, if present, prior to making the diagnosis.

Pharmacologic treatment for RBD is limited. The goal of treatment should be to reduce or eliminate the number of dream enactments that occur.[6] Clonazepam was the first medication used that had significant efficacy in the treatment of RBD with a reduction in RBD symptoms in 87% of patients.[17] The use of clonazepam may act by reducing the number of violent dreams, which can lead to a reduction in dream enactment in bed. A dosage range between 0.25 mg and 4 mg has been shown by to be efficacious. Because of the potential adverse effects of clonazepam in the elderly, the lowest efficacious dose should be chosen.[18]

Melatonin is the only medication that has been shown to restore muscle atonia during REM sleep. Melatonin has been shown to be effective in reducing the RBD frequency also. Doses between 3 mg and 15 mg (with an average dose of 6 mg) have been used with good efficacy and tolerability.[3,8,19] Because of the safety profile, melatonin may be used as the first agent in elderly patients.

Other classes of medications have been studied in RBD, but none have shown as much efficacy as clonazepam and melatonin. These include melatonergic agents, cannabidiol, and dopamine agents.[7,20] Acetylcholinesterase inhibitors such as donepezil and rivastigmine show promise, but more research is needed to validate these small studies.[21] Finally, there is some evidence to suggest that other benzodiazepines, such as temazepam, triazolam, and alprazolam, can be as effective as clonazepam.[20] Medications used to treat alpha-synucleinopathies (ie, Parkinson disease, multisystem atrophy disorder) do not diminish the frequency of RBD, as they focus on different pathways and mechanisms in the brain that do not interact with the areas affected with RBD.

As neurodegeneration progresses, the frequency and intensity of RBD can worsen. Therefore, treatment of RBD should focus on frequency of events and safety of the patient and bed partner. The goal of treatment is not to necessarily eliminate all abnormal movements during REM. There may continue to be evidence of REM without atonia (ie, mumbling, talking while asleep, and slight movements of extremities). The focus of treatment is to diminish the number of events that the patient has while also decreasing the severity of those behaviors. This will help ensure a safer environment for the patient and bed partner.[22]

Prognosis

Delayed emergence of a neurodegenerative disorder is common in men 50 years of age and older. It is now well established that RBD has been linked to the alpha synucleinopathies.[23] Up to 90.9% of patients with idiopathic RBD may ultimately develop a neurodegenerative disorder over a longitudinal follow-up.[24] It has been reported that RBD can precede the neurodegenerative process by up to 25 years. The risk for developing neurologic disease over the first 2 to 5 years is approximately 15% to 35%. This risk increases to 41% to 90.5% on follow-up between 12 and 25 years.[24] In patients with known established neurodegenerative disease, the prevalence of RBD was: 58% to 65% in Parkinson disease, 50% in Lewy-body dementia, and 68% to 90% in multisystem atrophy.[15,22,25] Patients with these conditions should be specifically asked about DEB and treated, given the risk of violent behavior.

OTHER PARASOMNIAS

The International Classification of Sleep Disorders categorizes parasomnias into 3 major categories: NREM-related parasomnias, REM-related parasomnias, and other parasomnias. However, some parasomnias overlap and may have a mixture of states.[1]

NREM-related parasomnias include disorders of arousal (eg, confusional arousals, sleepwalking, and sleep terrors), and sleep-related eating disorder (SRED). Disorders of arousal occur during partial arousals from slow wave (N3) sleep and are more commonly seen in children but can be present (up to 4%–5%) in older adults.[26,27] Treatment is often unnecessary, and reassurance to patients and families should be provided along with ensuring safety. Focus on prevention by eliminating exacerbating factors such as sleep deprivation, sedative use, or sleep disorders that may cause sleep instability may be helpful.[28] SRED consists of episodes of amnestic nocturnal sleepwalking associated with compulsive eating behavior, often of unusual food items (eg, soap, raw meat, dog food) and can have metabolic consequences including weight gain and poor glucose control. SRED is a parasomnia and should be distinguished from nocturnal eating syndrome, in which the patient is fully awake. SRED is generally most common in those with eating disorders, but a few case reports of SRED in patients with Parkinson disease have been reported.[29–31] Treatment includes management of underlying sleep disorders and ensuring safety of individuals. Medications that are associated with this condition, such as zolpidem and olanzapine, should be discontinued when possible. Dopamine agonists, SSRIs, and topiramate have been reported as pharmacologic treatment options.[32]

REM-related parasomnias include RBD, recurrent isolated sleep paralysis, and nightmare disorder. Sleep paralysis is elicited during awakening from REM sleep and is an example of state dissociation. It is common in narcolepsy but occurs often in isolation in the general population, usually in adolescence. Treatment typically involves reducing stressors and reassurance.[3] Nightmare disorder usually occurs in younger children but can be present in adults, particularly in the setting of trauma and post-traumatic stress disorder (PTSD). The best treatment for nightmare disorder is image rehearsal therapy, but lucid dreaming therapy and self-exposure therapy have also been reported. For PTSD-related nightmares, prazosin is an effective pharmacologic treatment option.[33]

CLINICS CARE POINTS

- REM behavior disorder is a REM parasomnia that should be screened for with an overnight in-laboratory polysomnography in patients having dream enactment.

- Idiopathic REM behavior disorder is a diagnosis associated with the alpha synucleopathies which may have a prodromal period of ten or more years.
- Treatment of REM behavior disorder consists of creating a safe sleeping environment as well as the addition of medications (eg, clonazepam and melatonin) to reduce the frequency of events.
- A thorough review of the patient's history is necessary to evaluate for secondary causes of REM behavior disorder (eg, medications and sleep disordered breathing).
- NREM parasomnias occur less commonly in older adults and are not associated with development of a neurodegenerative disorder.

DISCLOSURE

The authors have nothing to disclose.

REFERENCES

1. Medicine AAoS. International classification of sleep disorders. American Academy of Sleep Medicine. 3rd edition 2014.
2. Cooke JR, Ancoli-Israel S. Normal and abnormal sleep in the elderly. Handb Clin Neurol 2011;98:653–65.
3. Kryger MH, Roth T, Dement WC. Principles and practice of sleep medicine. 6th edition. Philadelphia, PA: Elsevier; 2017.
4. Bliwise DL. Sleep in normal aging and dementia. Sleep 1993;16(1):40–81.
5. Feinsilver SH, Hernandez AB. Sleep in the elderly: unanswered questions. Clin Geriatr Med 2017;33(4):579–96.
6. Boeve BF. REM sleep behavior disorder: updated review of the core features, the REM sleep behavior disorder-neurodegenerative disease association, evolving concepts, controversies, and future directions. Ann N Y Acad Sci 2010;1184:15–54.
7. Iranzo A. Parasomnias and sleep-related movement disorders in older adults. Sleep Med Clin 2018;13(1):51–61.
8. Rodriguez CL, Jaimchariyatam N, Budur K. Rapid eye movement sleep behavior disorder: a review of the literature and update on current concepts. Chest 2017;152(3):650–62.
9. Kang SH, Yoon IY, Lee SD, et al. REM sleep behavior disorder in the Korean elderly population: prevalence and clinical characteristics. Sleep 2013;36(8):1147–52.
10. Ju YE, Larson-Prior L, Duntley S. Changing demographics in REM sleep behavior disorder: possible effect of autoimmunity and antidepressants. Sleep Med 2011;12(3):278–83.
11. Berry RB, Brooks R, Gamaldo C, et al. AASM scoring manual updates for 2017 (Version 2.4). J Clin Sleep Med 2017;13(5):665–6.
12. Boeve BF, Molano JR, Ferman TJ, et al. Validation of the Mayo Sleep Questionnaire to screen for REM sleep behavior disorder in a community-based sample. J Clin Sleep Med 2013;9(5):475–80.
13. Available at: http://www.mayoclinic.org/pdfs/MSQ-copyrightfinal.pdf.
14. Li SX, Wing YK, Lam SP, et al. Validation of a new REM sleep behavior disorder questionnaire (RBDQ-HK). Sleep Med 2010;11(1):43–8.
15. Gagnon JF, Bedard MA, Fantini ML, et al. REM sleep behavior disorder and REM sleep without atonia in Parkinson's disease. Neurology 2002;59(4):585–9.

16. Iranzo A, Santamaria J. Severe obstructive sleep apnea/hypopnea mimicking REM sleep behavior disorder. Sleep 2005;28(2):203–6.

17. Olson EJ, Boeve BF, Silber MH. Rapid eye movement sleep behaviour disorder: demographic, clinical and laboratory findings in 93 cases. Brain 2000;123(Pt 2): 331–9.

18. McCarter SJ, Boswell CL, St Louis EK, et al. Treatment outcomes in REM sleep behavior disorder. Sleep Med 2013;14(3):237–42.

19. Kunz D, Bes F. Melatonin as a therapy in REM sleep behavior disorder patients: an open-labeled pilot study on the possible influence of melatonin on REM-sleep regulation. Mov Disord 1999;14(3):507–11.

20. Zhang F, Niu L, Liu X, et al. Rapid eye movement sleep behavior disorder and neurodegenerative diseases: an update. Aging Dis 2020;11(2):315–26.

21. Ringman JM, Simmons JH. Treatment of REM sleep behavior disorder with donepezil: a report of three cases. Neurology 2000;55(6):870–1.

22. Boeve BF, Silber MH, Ferman TJ. REM sleep behavior disorder in Parkinson's disease and dementia with Lewy bodies. J Geriatr Psychiatry Neurol 2004;17(3): 146–57.

23. McCarter SJ, St Louis EK, Boeve BF. REM sleep behavior disorder and REM sleep without atonia as an early manifestation of degenerative neurological disease. Curr Neurol Neurosci Rep 2012;12(2):182–92.

24. St Louis EK, Boeve BF. REM sleep behavior disorder: diagnosis, clinical Implications, and future directions. Mayo Clin Proc 2017;92(11):1723–36.

25. Plazzi G, Corsini R, Provini F, et al. REM sleep behavior disorders in multiple system atrophy. Neurology 1997;48(4):1094–7.

26. Crisp AH. The sleepwalking/night terrors syndrome in adults. Postgrad Med J 1996;72(852):599–604.

27. Mahowald MW, Bornemann MC, Schenck CH. Parasomnias. Semin Neurol 2004; 24(3):283–92.

28. Fleetham JA, Fleming JA. Parasomnias. CMAJ 2014;186(8):E273–80.

29. Auger RR. Sleep-related eating disorders. Psychiatry (Edgmont) 2006;3(11): 64–70.

30. Kaur H, Jahngir MU, Siddiqui JH. Sleep-related eating disorder in a patient with Parkinson's disease. Cureus 2018;10(9):e3345.

31. Sobreira Neto MA, Pereira MA, Sobreira ES, et al. Sleep-related eating disorder in two patients with early-onset Parkinson's disease. Eur Neurol 2011;66(2):106–9.

32. Schenck CH, Hurwitz TD, Bundlie SR, et al. Sleep-related eating disorders: polysomnographic correlates of a heterogeneous syndrome distinct from daytime eating disorders. Sleep 1991;14(5):419–31.

33. Morgenthaler TI, Auerbach S, Casey KR, et al. Position paper for the treatment of nightmare disorder in adults: an American Academy of Sleep Medicine position paper. J Clin Sleep Med 2018;14(6):1041–55.

Moving?

Make sure your subscription moves with you!

To notify us of your new address, find your **Clinics Account Number** (located on your mailing label above your name), and contact customer service at:

Email: journalscustomerservice-usa@elsevier.com

800-654-2452 (subscribers in the U.S. & Canada)
314-447-8871 (subscribers outside of the U.S. & Canada)

Fax number: 314-447-8029

Elsevier Health Sciences Division
Subscription Customer Service
3251 Riverport Lane
Maryland Heights, MO 63043

*To ensure uninterrupted delivery of your subscription, please notify us at least 4 weeks in advance of move.

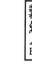

Printed and bound by CPI Group (UK) Ltd, Croydon, CR0 4YY

03/10/2024

01040401-0012